An Outline of Urology

An Outline of
Urology

D. E. Sturdy MS, FRCS

Consultant Surgeon, The Royal Gwent Hospital, Newport

Bristol
1986

Published under the Wright imprint by
IOP Publishing Limited,
Techno House, Redcliffe Way,
Bristol BS1 6NX, England

*British Library Cataloguing in
Publication Data*

Sturdy, D. E.
  An outline of urology
  1. Genito-urinary organs—Diseases
  I. Title
  616.6   RC871

  ISBN 0 7236 0885 7

By the same author
  Essentials of Urology
  Bristol, Wright, 1974

Typeset by Activity Limited,
Salisbury, Wiltshire, England

Printed in Great Britain by
Henry Ling Ltd, The Dorset Press, Dorchester

Preface

The purpose of this book is to give clinical surgical students an outline of diagnosis and management of disease of the genito-urinary system. With this in view, descriptive text has been curtailed to the minimum and liberal use has been made of line diagrams and radiographs. Over the past decade methods of investigation of the urinary tract have developed rapidly and it is essential that medical students should have a working knowledge of the newer techniques. The basic format of the book is a brief description of the pathology and clinical features of urological disease with a more detailed appraisal of diagnostic methods employed and a report on the current treatment of any particular urological condition. The book should be useful to the clinical student and junior house officer as a ready reminder of present-day urological practice and as a volume for reading in preparation for examinations in surgery.

I am indebted to Dr Glas Griffiths and Dr Richard Harding, of the Department of Radiology of the Royal Gwent Hospital, for providing radiographic material and isotope scans. Mr Geoff Lyth has revised many of my line diagrams and prepared six new sketches. Mr Nigel Pearce and staff of the Department of Medical Illustration, Newport Hospitals, have been extremely helpful in reproducing radiographs, scans and line diagrams. My secretary, Mrs Sharon Smith, has shown inestimable patience and industry in typing the manuscript. I am extremely grateful to her and to John Wright & Sons for their advice and co-operation in producing the proofs and publishing this Outline textbook on urological surgery.

D.E.S.

Contents

1

General considerations

• A. Applied Anatomy of the Urinary Tract

The Kidney
    The kidneys are retroperitoneal organs lying opposite the 12th thoracic and upper three lumbar vertebrae, the left kidney being 2–3 cm higher in position than the right. The right kidney has the 12th rib in posterior relation to its upper third, whilst the 11th and 12th ribs lie behind the upper half of the left kidney (*Fig.* 1.1). Trauma, haematuria and radiological fractures of the 11th or 12th ribs indicate renal contusion or laceration. The relations of the structures in the renal hilum from the front to back are the vein, the artery and the renal pelvis–VAP (*Fig.* 1.2). The renal pelvis is accessible from the back or laterally, whilst an anterior approach is used for exposure of the vessels in the renal hilum.

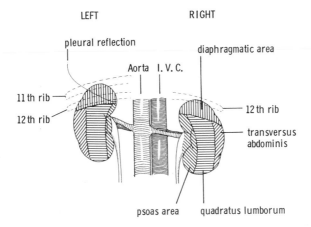

Fig. 1.1 Posterior relations of the kidneys (note pleural reflection behind upper pole of the left kidney).

The Ureter
    The intra-abdominal ureter runs along the tips of the transverse processes of L2, L3, L4 and L5 lumbar vertebrae, crossing into the pelvis at the mid-point of the sacro-iliac joint, deviating laterally towards the ischial spine and then

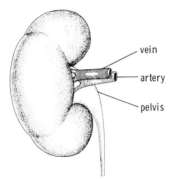

Fig. 1.2 Relations of the structures in the hilum of the kidney viewed from the front.

ascending forwards and medially to the base of the bladder. Radio-opaque calculi must be looked for along this line (*Fig*. 1.7). In the female the terminal 2 cm of the ureter are closely related to the vaginal fornix, especially on the left side where it may be at risk during gynaecological and pelvic surgical operations. The normal ureter exhibits three sites of natural narrowing—the pelvi-ureteric junction A, the bony pelvic brim A_1 and within the bladder wall B (*Fig*. 1.3).

Calculi within the ureter tend to lodge and ureteric strictures tend to occur at these three sites. Medial deviation of the abdominal ureter may indicate a caecal or ascending colon tumour on the right and a descending or pelvic colon tumour on the left. Medial deviation and obstruction of both ureters may be due to fibrosis, as in tuberculosis or retroperitoneal fibrosis. Lateral displacement of one or both ureters within the abdomen is diagnostic of a midline retroperitoneal lesion such as an aortic aneurysm or retroperitoneal tumour.

The Bladder and Prostate

In the neonatal period and infancy the urinary bladder is mainly abdominal in position and clothed with peritoneum over the upper two-thirds of its external surface; it is often easily palpated on abdominal examination. The bladder descends into the bony pelvis in childhood and in the adult only the upper one-third anteriorly and the posterior two-thirds (recto-vesical pouch) are covered with peritoneum. Trauma such as a pelvic fracture usually damages the extraperitoneal surface of the bladder (*Fig*. 5.4), except when the bladder is full of urine. The prostate gland and pubo-prostatic ligaments invest the lower trigone, bladder neck and first part of the urethra, anchoring these structures at fixed points, the rest of the bladder being mobile and contractile. Pelvic fractures produce a urethral rupture by a sheering rotational force on this fixed point of the prostatic urethra (*Fig*. 1.4). The lateral lobes of the prostate gland are easily palpable by digital examination of the rectum. Eighty per cent of carcinomas arise in the postero-lateral aspect of the prostate gland and should be accessible to diagnosis by a rectal examination.

The Urethra

The male urethra is 18–20 cm long and exhibits three points of natural narrowing—the bladder neck C, the perineal membrane (at the apex of the prostate gland) C_1 and the external urinary meatus D (*Fig*. 1.3). The narrowest point in the

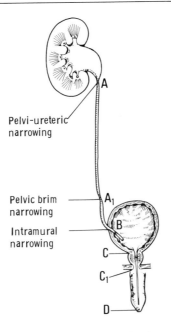

Pelvi-ureteric
narrowing

Pelvic brim
narrowing

Intramural
narrowing

Fig. 1.3 Points of natural narrowing in the urinary tract.

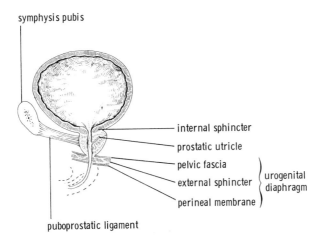

symphysis pubis

internal sphincter

prostatic utricle

pelvic fascia

external sphincter

perineal membrane

urogenital
diaphragm

puboprostatic ligament

Fig. 1.4 Sagittal section of bladder, prostate gland and sphincters.

male urethra is at the perineal membrane, with the narrowest segment in the terminal 1 cm of the urethra within the glans penis. An instrument which negotiates the terminal urethra will usually pass into the bladder without difficulty. Strictures of the urethra due to infection, such as venereal disease, or due to instrumental damage tend to occur at these points of natural narrowing within the male urethra.

Lymphatic Drainage

The scrotum, penis and penile urethra as far as the perineal membrane will drain into the associated inguinal lymph nodes. The testis and cord will drain into the external iliac and para-aortic lymph nodes. The prostate, bladder and pelvic ureter will drain into the internal iliac and para-aortic nodes. The kidney and upper ureter will drain into nodes along the vena cava and to the para-aortic nodes (*Fig.* 1.5). Malignant tumours of various sections of the genito-urinary tract may be expected to metastasize to the appropriate group of regional lymph nodes.

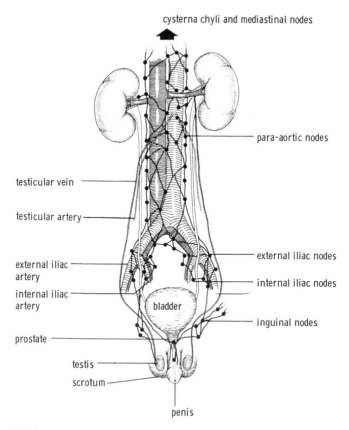

Fig. 1.5 Lymphatic drainage and arterial supply of the genito-urinary tract.

● **B. Basic Renal Physiology**

The functional unit of the kidney is the nephron, each kidney containing one million units. The head of the nephron in the renal cortex is the glomerulus, which acts as a filter for a perfusate of protein-free plasma to pass from the glomerular capillaries into Bowman's capsule. The capsular space within the glomerulus is continuous with the renal tubule, which is constructed in three functional segments—the proximal convoluted tubule, the loop of Henle and the distal convoluted tubule—each with its own specific function. The perfusate passes into collecting tubules and collecting ducts (*Fig.* 1.6), which discharge urine

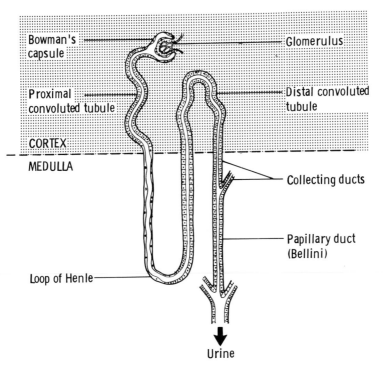

Fig. 1.6 The nephron.

into the renal calices via the papillary ducts (ducts of Bellini). Glomerular function separates an ultra-filtrate from the circulating plasma in the glomerular capillaries. Filtration pressure drives the ultra-filtrate onwards through the renal tubules, where selective reabsorption and selective secretion modify the concentration of the filtrate to produce urine.

The kidneys have two functions in human physiology—regulatory and endocrine.

Regulatory Functions.
1. Regulation of composition of body fluids by a complex combination of filtration, reabsorption and secretion of the solutes sodium, potassium,

chloride, bicarbonate, phosphate, calcium, glucose, amino acids, urea and uric acid.
2.   Maintenance of acid–base balance by bicarbonate reabsorption and excretion of excess acid in the urine.
3.   Regulation of volume of extra-cellular fluid by control of excretion of sodium chloride.
4.   Extraction of a number of amino acids for the synthesis of ammonia.
5.   In starvation, the kidneys release glucose into the circulation.

Endocrine Functions
1.   Secretion of renin—neuro-hormonal regulating mechanism which, with angiotensin and aldosterone, controls body water and sodium content, potassium balance and arterial blood pressure.
2.   Secretion of erythropoietin involved in normal replacement of red blood cells and for accelerated erythropoiesis in stress states such as haemorrhage, altitude exposure and haemolysis.
3.   Secretion of prostaglandins—affect smooth muscle contraction in the uterus and gastro-intestinal tract, increase salt and water clearance by the kidney, increase thyroid function and inhibition of lipolysis.
4.   Synthesis of 1,25-dihydroxycholecalciferol from vitamin D—important in the regulation of calcium transportation in the body.

The functions of the various sections of the nephron are complex and interrelated.
1.   *The glomerulus* has two simplified basic functions:
       Regulatory: Acts as a filter.
       Endocrine: Site of secretion of renin, erythropoietin, prostaglandins and breakdown of vitamin D.
2.   *The proximal convoluted tubule*—reabsorption of main bulk of solutes in ultra-filtrate.
3.   *The loop of Henle*—maintains osmolarity of the fluid and releases sodium chloride.
4.   *The distal convoluted tubule, the collecting tubules and collecting ducts*—involved in concentration or dilution of urine and in fine regulation of sodium excretion, in secretion of hydrogen ions and in regulation of urinary potassium concentration.

Tests of Renal Function
       The use of haematological and biochemical methods for estimating renal function has been largely superseded by DTPA radio-isotope scanning and differential renal function scans (p. 14). The scan is an invasive technique but does not involve the use of iodine-based contrast medium, thus eliminating the problem of iodine sensitivity.
       Clearances of the endogenous markers urea and creatinine are useful indicators of renal function. The urea level (normal 2·3–6·9 mmol/l) is elevated with impaired renal function but may also be raised in other conditions, e.g. dehydration, intestinal haemorrhage and cardiac failure. The normal blood creatinine level is 50–120 μmol/l, often elevated in failing or obstructed kidneys. The creatinine clearance test is used on occasions for estimating renal function. Blood and urine samples are assessed for creatinine content over

a period of 24 hours in a fasting patient. A delay in clearance of creatinine from blood into the urine is indicative of impairment of renal function.

● **C. Clinical Examination of the Genito-urinary Patient**

Symptomatology
> The four principal complaints are:
1. Pain in the kidney and ureter—renal pain: ureteric colic.
2. Pain on passing urine—dysuria.
3. Blood in the urine—haematuria.
4. Disorder in passage of urine—frequency: incontinence: difficulty or inability to micturate.

> The characteristics of these complaints are:
1. Renal pain:
   A dull boring ache in the loin with anterior radiation under the costal margin and often aggravated by jolting movements such as car journeys or jogging.
2. Ureteric colic:
   The most violent pain a human can experience: occurring in waves, associated with clinical shock and vomiting and often referred to the groin or testis in the male and the groin, vagina or labia in the female.
3. Bladder pain:
   Dull and located in the suprapubic area: with dysuria and frequency, indicates cystitis. Bladder pain in acute retention of urine is severe (bursting). The chronically distended bladder is painless.
4. Dysuria:
   Pain or discomfort passing urine: referred to the end of the penis in the male. Terminal dysuria indicates inflammation of the bladder neck or prostate gland. Dysuria is commonly accompanied by frequency.
5. Haematuria:
   Painful macroscopic bleeding indicates inflammation of the bladder or prostate. Tumours of the urothelium—painless haematuria. Large blood clots in the urine—bladder origin. Spindle-shaped clots with ureteric colic—renal origin (clot colic).
6. Frequency:
   A normal young adult micturates four to six times in 24 hr and not at all during sleep. Older patients may void seven or eight times during the day and once or twice at night. Nocturia refers to voiding in excess of two times during sleeping hours. Frequency is a prominent symptom in bladder outflow obstruction (prostatism). Frequency invariably accompanies dysuria in infection.
7. Incontinence:
   Involuntary loss of urine from the bladder. In urge incontinence the patient is unable to get to the toilet in time to empty the bladder. Prostatic patients may have terminal incontinence (dribbling) with loss of some residual urine

after the act of micturition is complete. Stress incontinence on straining, coughing or sneezing occurs in the female patient with uterine prolapse. True incontinence appears in patients with congenital or acquired neurogenic bladder lesions—no control by the patient over the act of voiding. Overflow incontinence occurs in the chronically obstructed bladder.

8.   Difficulty with micturition:

Encountered in patients with bladder outflow obstruction or urethral strictures. Patients complain of difficulty in starting, a 'thin' or poor stream during the act and terminal dribbling or incontinence at the end of the act. Complete inability to void urine occurs in acute retention of urine.

Physical Examination

Physical examination of the genito-urinary patient must include a general medical assessment combined with a specific examination of the genito-urinary system.

General Physical Examination

1.   Cardiovascular and pulmonary systems with recording of blood pressure.
2.   Conjunctivae, palms of hands and finger nails for evidence of anaemia.
3.   Tongue inspected and breath smelt to detect the mawkish odour of uraemia.

Examination of the Genito-urinary System

1.   Smell:

Uriniferous odour of patients' underclothes, indicating incontinence.

2.   Inspection:

From the front, side and back with the patient standing and recumbent.

In infants, inspection is the most reliable method of spotting an abdominal mass.

Bulging in the loins or a midline suprapubic swelling.

3.   Palpation:

Enlargement of the kidneys, liver, bladder and intra-abdominal masses.

The kidney must be enlarged two or three times its normal size to be bimanually palpable; the left kidney is palpated from the patient's left side.

The distended bladder is visible and palpable in most patients but difficulty may arise in obesity.

4.   Percussion:

Size of enlarged kidney and bladder—dull to percussion.

Abdominal ascites—shifting dullness.

5.   Auscultation:

Over the aorta and renal vessels.

A bruit indicates an aortic aneurysm, stenosis of the renal artery or renal arteriovenous fistula.

6.   External genitalia:

Easily accessible for inspection: excoriation and brown discoloration of skin in incontinent patients.

Prepuce, glans penis and external meatus inspected for meatal stenosis, phimosis, hypospadias and penile tumours.

Testis, epididymis and cord inspected for cysts or tumours.
Groins examined for lymphadenopathy or hernia.
Scrotal swelling—a hernia, hydrocele or tumour. A hernia is reducible; a hydrocele transilluminates in a darkened room.

7. Rectal examination:
Mandatory in the male.
Excludes pathology within the rectum.
Determines size, contour and consistency of the prostate gland.
Fixation of the rectal mucosa, obliteration of the median sulcus between the two lobes of the prostate and a hard rock-like gland—diagnostic of prostatic carcinoma.

8. Pelvic examination
Mandatory in the female.

● **D. Investigation of the Urinary Tract**

The genito-urinary tract can be accurately and completely assessed by a combination of haematological, bacteriological, biochemical, radiographic and endoscopic examination.

Urine
1. The end product of renal function.
2. Volume voided at each micturition—normally 250–300 ml.
3. Volume excreted in 24 hr—average 1200–1500 ml.
4. Concentration of urine sample (hygrometer)—normally 1010.
5. Reaction of urine (pH)—litmus test—acid red: alkaline blue.

Colour of Urine
1. Dark golden brown—bile.
2. Cloudy with white deposit
Phosphates (clears on acidification).
Infection of urine.
3. Pink or port wine—blood (beware betroot or rhubarb).
4. Deep red—phenolphthalein.
5. Greenish tinge—methylene blue: de Witts pills.
6. Normal yellow urine becoming deep red on standing—porphyrinuria.

Smell of Urine
Ammoniacal or 'fishy' odour—infection with *Bacillus, Proteus* or *Pyocyaneus*.

Ward Testing—Labstix
Urine may be tested for bile, blood, protein, ketones.

Laboratory Tests of Midstream Specimen
1. Red blood cells—microscopic haematuria—pathology of urinary tract (exception menstruating females).
2. White blood cells—over 5 cells/mm^2—infection.
3. Chemical constituents—oxalates, phosphates, cystine.

4.   Bacilli—*Mycobacterium tuberculosis*.
5.   Cytology—malignant cells of urothelial origin.
6.   Culture:
           Infective organisms—sensitivity of organisms determined for a range
           of antibiotics. Lowenstein culture for *M. tuberculosis*.
Note:
           Examination of the urine is undertaken on a midstream specimen after
           cleansing the prepuce and glans penis in the male and swabbing the vulva in
           the female. In neonates and infants, suprapubic aspiration of the bladder may
           be necessary to obtain a clean sample of urine.

Blood
1.   Haemoglobin estimation:
           Male 14 g per cent.
           Female 12·5 g per cent.
2.   White cell count:
           Elevated polymorphonuclear count in infection.
3.   Erythrocyte sedimentation rate:
           Normally under 12 mm/hr—non-specific indicator of pathology.
4.   Blood urea. Normally 2·3–6·9 mmol/1—elevated in renal failure and
           obstructive uropathy,
5.   Serum creatinine. Normally 50–120 μmol/1—elevated in obstructive
           uropathy.
6.   Serum calcium. Normally 2·15–2·60 mmol/1—elevated in hyperpara-
           thyroidism.
7.   Serum alkaline phosphatase. Normally 30–115 IU/1—elevated in skeletal
           metastases.
8.   Prostatic acid phosphatase. Normally 0–4·0 IU/1—elevated in carci-
           noma of the prostate.
9.   Culture. Positive in septicaemic patients.

Renal Function Tests
           The only test of value in clinical urology is the creatinine clearance test
(p. 6). Renal function and differential function of each kidney are assessed by
renal nuclear imaging (p. 14).

Radiological Investigation of the Urinary Tract
           Accurate diagnosis of pathological lesions in the urinary tract is nearly
always possible by a combination of invasive and non-invasive techniques, some
of which have a therapeutic application.

Plain Films of the Abdomen
The film must include the lower ribs, the bony pelvis and the external genitalia.
The plain film is examined for position, shape and size of the kidneys, evidence of
calculi or calcification and the presence of skeletal metastases. Interpretation of a
plain abdominal X-ray is illustrated in *Fig.* 1.7.

Excretion Urography (Intravenous Urography): IVU
A routine examination in urological practice After 12 hr limitation of fluids,

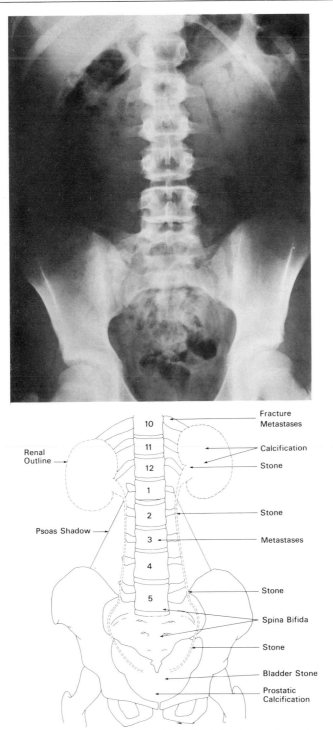

Fig. 1.7 Interpretation of a plain abdominal radiograph.

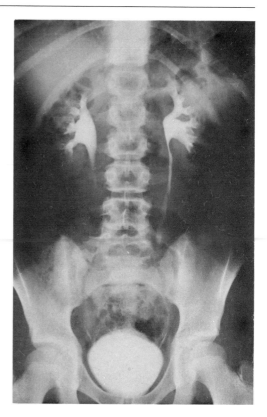

50 ml of iodine contrast medium is administered intravenously and films taken at 5, 10, 20 and 30 min. In delayed excretion films are taken at 1–2 and up to 24 hr after the injection. The high dose technique uses 100 ml of dye in a single bolus injection. The excreted dye collects in the bladder (cystogram phase) and a post-micturition film will demonstrate the presence or absence of residual urine. The symptoms of iodine sensitivity vary from mild nausea, vomiting, itching and urticarial rashes to laryngeal spasm, hypotension and cardiac arrest.

Contraindications to IVU
1.   Positive history of iodine sensitivity.
2.   General tendency to allergic reactions.
3.   Pregnancy.
4.   Renal and liver failure.
5.   Multiple myeloma.

Reading an IVU (*Fig.* 1.7 and *Fig.* 1.8).
Inspect the preliminary plain abdominal film and look for:
1.   Bony abnormalities—spina bifida, fractures, metastases.
2.   Renal outlines and edge of the psoas muscle.
3.   Calcification:
         In renal cortex.
         In midline—aortic aneurysm.
4.   Calculus:
         In renal area.

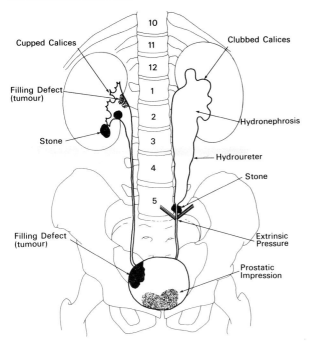

Fig. 1.8 Interpretation of an IVU.

       In ureter along lines of transverse process.
       In bony pelvis or midline (bladder stone).
    Inspect the complete range of IVU films, in order, and look for:

1. Position of kidneys and renal contour.
2. Renal calices, cupped or clubbed.
3. Renal pelvis for distension and irregular outline due to tumour or stone.
4. The ureter for dilatation or displacement.
5. The bladder for displacement, intrinsic filling defect.
6. Diverticulum.
7. The post-micturition film for residual urine and 'prostatic impression'.

Note:

    Unilateral hydroureter—obstruction may be extrinsic (pressure from without by an abdominal or pelvic tumour), intrinsic (fibrosis or tumour) or within the lumen (calculus). Bilateral hydroureter—bladder outlet or urethral obstruction (prostatic hypertrophy or carcinoma, urethral stricture).

Retrograde Ureterography

A catheter is introduced via a cystoscope into the lower ureter and contrast medium is injected retrogradely up the ureter. Combined with image intensification and video-recording, the technique provides a dynamic record of the contractile function of the ureter and renal pelvis.

Antegrade Pyelography
Investigation of hydronephrosis. A fine needle is introduced percutaneously from the loin into the distended renal pelvis. Intrapelvic pressure is recorded and pyelography demonstrates the site of obstruction.

Cystourethrography
Contrast medium introduced into the bladder via a catheter which is removed. During voiding contrast may be seen refluxing up the ureter and the urethra is delineated during voiding. In infants the investigation is undertaken under a general anaesthetic and a compression cystourethrogram is obtained.

Urethrography
Retrograde introduction of dye into the male urethra via a catheter. The technique is employed in investigation of urethral strictures.

Radioisotope Scans
Two methods of investigation are available—diuresis renography and static renal scanning.

Diuresis Renography
Technetium-labelled DTPA is administered intravenously and counts in each loin are recorded on a gamma camera. The radioisotope is actively secreted by the renal tubules, giving quantitative data of function of each kidney. After 20 min a diuretic is administered, and a rapid fall in counts indicates no obstruction whilst a rising static count indicates stasis or obstruction to the kidney (*Fig.* 1.9). Vesico-ureteric reflux can be detected by this investigation.

Static Renal Scan
Technetium-labelled DMSA is selectively retained in the renal cortex, and the examination is of value in demonstrating the size and position of the kidneys and in locating parenchymal defects such as cysts or tumours (*Fig.* 1.10).

Note:
> Radioisotope scans have a low radiation exposure and are not subject to adverse sensitivity reactions.

Ultrasonography
A non-invasive investigation. Ultrasound is a form of energy consisting of mechanical vibrations at a frequency too high to be detected by the human ear. The ultrasound waves rebound from the structures within the body and echoes from solid, semi-solid and fluid components vary in intensity producing a grey-scale recording.

Ultrasound of the Kidney
Renal parenchyma—echo poor.
Renal pelvis—echogenic (*Fig.* 1.11).

Ultrasound of the Bladder
Fluid-filled bladder—echo free.
Bladder tumour—echo poor.

Ultrasound of the Prostate
The ultrasound probe is inserted into the rectum or urethra. A prostatic scan can

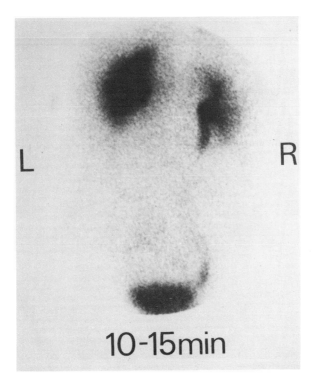

Fig. 1.9 DTPA isotope scan of a normal right and an obstructed left kidney. (*Note*: right and left kidneys reversed compared with an IVU.)

differentiate between tumour, hypertrophy and prostatitis, and is used for staging prostatic tumours and assessing their response to treatment.

Selective Renal Angiography
A fine catheter is inserted percutaneously into the femoral artery (Seldinger method) and guided under X-ray control into the renal artery or its branches. Anatomy of the renal arteries is visualized and renal tumours are diagnosed by this examination (*Fig.* 2.21).

Future Development
Digital vascular imaging (DVI) introduced as a computer-based method of angiography.

Computerized Axial Tomography (CT Scan)
The internal organs are scanned in serial planes (tomography) and the resultant images collated by computer. Images of the size, shape and inter-related positions of the internal organs are produced, with localization of space-occupying lesions within and between the organs.

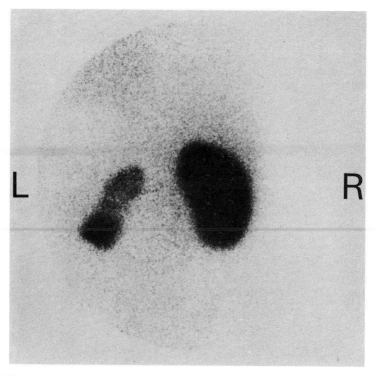

Fig. 1.10 DMSA scan of a normal right and a small scarred left kidney.

Inferior Vena Cavogram

Percutaneous puncture of the femoral vein and injection of contrast medium into the vena cava may demonstrate a blockage, blood clot or tumour infiltration of the cava.

Lymphography

Contrast medium is injected into the lymphatic vessel on the dorsum of the foot and X-rays taken of the inguinal external iliac and para-aortic lymph nodes. The technique is used (*Fig*. 6.18) to demonstrate malignant metastatic deposits in these groups of nodes. Lymphography has been superseded by CT scanning in those centres where a CT scanner is available.

Therapeutic Application of Radiological Techniques

Renal Drainage

Obstructed kidneys are decompressed by percutaneous catheter nephrostomy (pigtail catheter) introduced under ultrasound guidance.

Renal Cysts

Cysts of the kidney may be drained and cured by a similar technique.

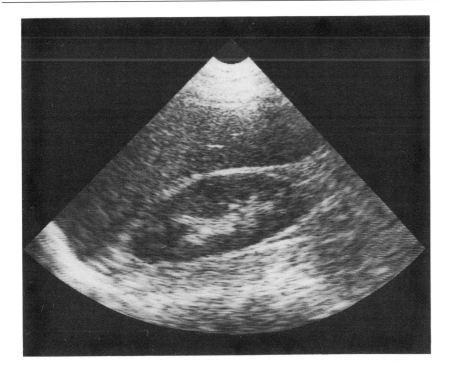

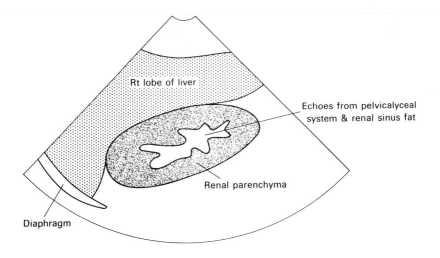

Fig. 1.11 Longitudinal ultrasound scan of a normal right kidney.

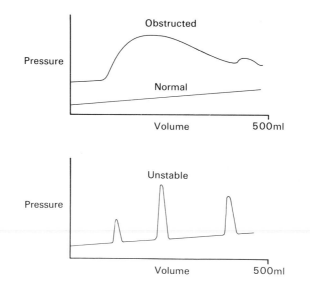

Fig. 1.12 Urodynamic studies of a normal, obstructed and unstable bladder.

Renal Stones
Small stones in the renal pelvis may be removed percutaneously under ultrasound guidance.

Tumour Embolization
Deliberate occlusion of a branch of the renal artery by embolic material introduced through a selectively positioned Seldinger catheter. The technique may be used for control of bleeding from the renal cortex, e.g. a haemangioma, or for the treatment of renal tumours in critically ill or elderly patients. The embolizing agents used are varied—gelatin sponge, human dura mater, steel coils, plastic or glass beads and detachable balloons.

Transluminal Angioplasty
Dilatation and stretching of a stenosis of the renal artery during selective angiography.

Lithotripsy
Disintegration of stones in renal pelvis by external high-frequency ultrasound (p. 62).

Investigation of Bladder Function
Investigations of bladder emptying (bladder outflow studies) are of two types:
Urinary flow rate studies.
Filling and voiding cystometry (urodynamics).

Urinary Flow Rate
A non-invasive method of determining whether a patient will benefit from

outflow tract surgery. The patient urinates without straining into a flow-meter which measures the rate of increase in volume of urine on voiding. In a normal male who voids 250–300 ml of urine the flow rate is in the region of 26 ml per s. In patients with significant outflow obstruction the flow rate is under 12 ml per s.

Urodynamic Studies

Following catheterization, the bladder is filled with saline at a constant rate and intravesical pressure measured by an electrode placed alongside the catheter. Abdominal pressure is measured by a similar catheter sited in the rectum. Filling cystometry records the pressure changes within the distending bladder. For the voiding phase of the investigation the catheter is removed from the bladder, the electrode left in situ and the pressure changes on voiding recorded. Urodynamic studies give an indication of function of the bladder during distension and contraction. Abnormalities of bladder function such as outflow obstruction, neurogenic instability and irregular detrusor activity (unstable bladder) are demonstrated by this technique (*Fig.* 1.12). By using contrast medium instead of saline, the urodynamic study can be combined with radiological screening of the lower urinary tract (video-cystometry).

Endoscopic Examination of the Urinary Tract

Cystourethroscopy

Cystourethroscopy allows direct examination of the interior of the bladder and urethra. Retrograde catheterization of the ureters, bladder biopsies and diathermy treatment of small lesions within the bladder can also be undertaken at cystourethroscopy. Examination of the lower urinary tract proceeds from the external meatus to the bladder neck (urethrocystoscopy). The bladder interior is inspected in a circular fashion, commencing at the fundus, where an air bubble is normally encountered, and ending at the bladder neck. Normal bladder urothelium is smooth, pale yellow with fine interwoven blood vessels, especially around the trigone. The ureteric orifices appear as crescentic slits or rounded openings flat on the bladder base or raised on small nipples. The intra-mural ureter can be seen as an oblique ridge leading down to the ureteric orifice. Another ridge, the interureteric bar, extends from one ureteric orifice to the other (*Fig.* 1.13). Endoscopically, the prostatic urethra is spindle-shaped and the verumontanum is seen in the midline posteriorly 2·5 cm below the bladder neck (*Fig.* 1.14). The normal bladder neck is circular. The anterior urethra is pale yellow in colour and has two points of narrowing—at the perineal membrane and at the external urinary meatus. It follows that if an instrument can negotiate the external urinary meatus it should pass readily into the bladder.

Nephroscopy

Examination of the interior of the renal pelvis and calices: used on occasions at open operation for removal of retained fragments of stones.

Future Development

Nephroscopes have been designed for inspection of the renal pelvis and stone extraction via the percutaneous route. The operating ureteroscope is introduced into the ureter via a cystoscope and used for ureteric biopsies and extraction of ureteric calculi.

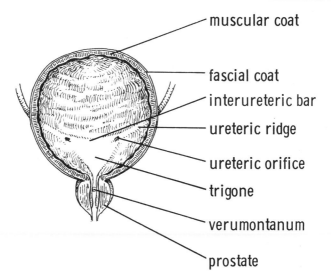

Fig. 1.13 Internal view of bladder, trigone and bladder neck.

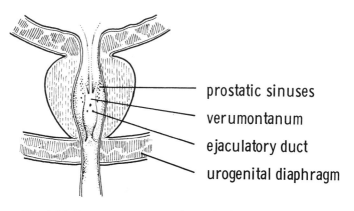

Fig. 1.14 Structures on posterior wall of prostatic urethra.

- ### E. Pre- and Postoperative Management of the Urological Patient

Preoperative Management

Urological patients, many of whom are elderly, require a general medical assessment combined with specific preparation of the urinary tract before operation.

General Assessment
1. Correction of anaemia: blood grouping.
2. Diagnosis and control of diabetes.

3.   Medical control of hypertension.
4.   Electrocardiograph for evidence of myocardial disease.
5.   Chest X-ray and preoperative physiotherapy.
6.   In undernourished patients—high calorie diet and vitamin therapy.
7.   Explanation of the operation proposed and boosting the patient's confidence in a successful outcome to the operative procedure.

Preparation of the Urinary Tract for Surgery
1.   Rehydration of the patient.
2.   Elimination of infection from the urinary tract with systemic antibiotics. In catheterized patients—anti-bacterial bladder washouts.
3.   Reversal of renal failure:
       Long-term catheterization with antibiotic cover in chronic renal failure.
       Nephrostomy drainage of obstructed kidney.
   The aim of these preoperative measures is to allow the urologist to operate on as fit a patient as possible and a patient with normal renal function and a sterile urinary tract.

Postoperative Management
   The two main problems in the patient after surgery on the urinary tract are haemorrhage and infection. The patient will also be subject to the hazards that exist after any surgical procedure.

Haemorrhage
Blood loss must be accurately measured and blood volume restored by transfusion. Prolonged hypotension, especially in the elderly, may cause renal ischaemia and failure, deep vein thrombosis, cerebral thrombosis and coronary artery occlusion.

Infection
Infection in the urinary tract, especially in obstructive uropathy, must be vigorously treated with antibiotics. Most patients after operation will have a catheter draining the urinary tract, and the tube is sometimes the source of infection. In the presence of an elevated temperature and pulse rate and bacteriological evidence of urinary infection, adequate antibiotic therapy is mandatory. After surgery all catheters and drainage tubes are managed on a 'closed' system of drainage in an attempt to eliminate the risk of introducing infection into the urinary tract.
   Apart from these specific postoperative measures, general management by routine physiotherapy and early ambulation are prescribed in the hope of preventing cardiac or pulmonary complications, phlebothrombosis and pulmonary embolism.

2

The kidney

Congenital Anomalies

Two types of congenital renal anomaly exist:

Developmental anomalies in the normally placed kidney (*Fig.* 2.1).
Anomaly in position or rotation of a fully developed kidney (*Fig.* 2.2).

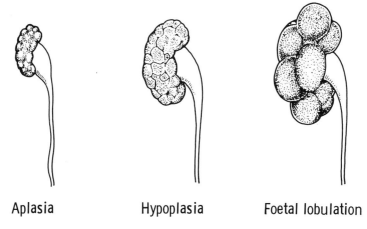

Aplasia   Hypoplasia   Foetal lobulation

Fig. 2.1 Anomalies in development of a normally positioned kidney.

The developing kidney has a lobulated contour and becomes reniform during the last 6 weeks of fetal life. Persistence of fetal lobulation in the adult has no functional significance. Renal agenesis (absence of kidney and ureter) is found in 1 per 400 patients. The contralateral kidney is hypertrophied and life expectancy is normal, provided the solitary kidney does not become obstructed or diseased. The aplastic kidney contains very few nephrons and is associated with a small contracted pelvis and ureter. The hypoplastic kidney is a miniature reproduction of the adult organ—it may become infected and pyelonephritic with hypertension. Radiologically, the hypoplastic kidney is small with a crenated outline and poor function on excretion urography. Nephrectomy is advocated for

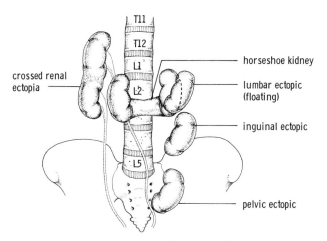

Fig. 2.2 Anomalies of renal position.

unilateral hypoplasia with infection and hypertension. In bilateral hypoplasia the outlook is poor, unless renal function and growth can be maintained to allow renal transplantation in childhood. A dysplastic kidney contains abnormal elements—fibrous tissue, cartilage and striated muscle. Such a kidney is frequently small, containing cysts, pyelonephritic and associated with hypertension. Unilateral dysplastic kidneys are removed by nephrectomy. Renal ultrasonography and renal isotope (DMSA) scans are the investigations of choice for detecting these anomalies (*Fig.* 1.10).

The kidney develops in the pelvis and moves cranially to reach its position on the posterior abdominal wall. Cranial migration may arrest at any point, giving rise to a pelvic, inguinal or lumbar ectopic kidney (*Fig.* 2.2). In the pelvis the kidney may be mistaken for a gynaecological tumour and in the inguinal region the kidney mimics a large bowel tumour. A variant of lumbar ectopic is the floating kidney, where the renal vessels are elongated with excessive mobility of the kidney. Diagnosis of an ectopic kidney is by ultrasound scan with absent echoes from the ipsilateral loin. An IVU confirms the diagnosis, and surgical treatment is only necessary if the ectopic kidney is infected or obstructed. In malrotation, the renal hilum lies in front of a vertically placed kidney and the upper ureter may be angulated. In a 'horseshoe kidney' the lower poles of the malrotated low-lying (lumbar ectopic) kidneys are joined by an isthmus of renal or fibrous tissue. Diagnosis is by an ultrasound scan, confirmed by an IVU in which the renal calices face anteriorly or medially towards the lumbar spine (*Fig.* 2.3). The ureters, crossing behind the isthmus, are frequently compressed and treatment consists of excision of the isthmus with release of the obstructed ureters. In crossed renal ectopia (very rare) both renal masses are found on one side of the abdomen (*Fig.* 2.4). One or other ureter has to cross behind the aorta and vena cava to reach the appropriate side of the bladder trigone.

Renal Cysts

Cystic spaces may occur in the renal parenchyma in a variety of conditions. Some are congenital (dysplastic) or traumatic in origin. Some are related to

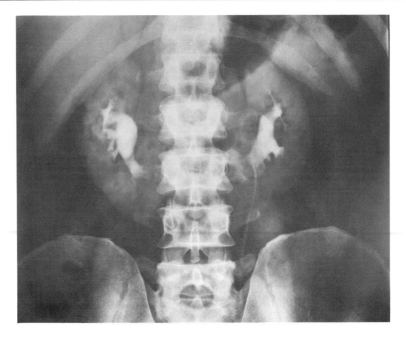

Fig. 2.3 IVU showing a horseshoe kidney.

chronic infection (medullary sponge kidney) and some are due to an obstruction of a calix (hydrocalicosis). Hydatid disease of the kidney, though very rare, may give rise to a cystic lesion in the parenchyma.

True cysts of the kidney, not associated with disease or obstruction and not connected with the renal calices and pelvis, are of three varieties (*Fig.* 2.5):
1. Solitary cyst.
2. Multicystic kidney.
3. Polycystic kidney.

Solitary Cyst
1. *Aetiology*:
    Unknown.
2. *Presentation*:
    Chance discovery by the patient: at routine clinical abdominal examination: at operative exploration of the abdomen.
3. *Complications*:
    Rupture—very rare occurrence.
    Infection—mimics a perinephric abscess.
    Haemorrhage—enlargement in size with pain and tenderness in loin.
4. *Diagnosis*:
    Differential diagnosis of a renal mass is between a renal cyst or a renal neoplasm. A protocol for differentiation between the two conditions is set out in *Fig.* 2.6. Ultrasonography demonstrates the cyst in most patients (*Fig.* 2.7).

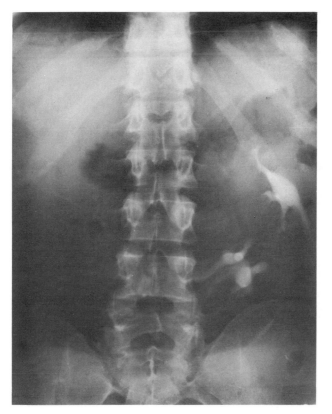

Fig. 2.4 IVU in a patient with crossed renal ectopia.

5. *Treatment*:
   Uncomplicated cyst in the elderly—no treatment.
   Younger patients—percutaneous cyst aspiration with ultrasound control.
   Rarely is surgical excision advised.

Multicystic Kidney

Multiple cysts are found in dysplastic functionless kidneys in infancy and childhood and are treated by nephrectomy. Multiple cysts may occur in an otherwise normal kidney. No treatment is indicated, unless one or two of the cysts enlarge—treated by percutaneous needle aspiration with ultrasound control.

Polycystic Kidney

In this condition the parenchyma of both kidneys is almost completely replaced by myriads of small tense cysts.

Incidence

1 in 4000 live births: associated with polycystic disease of liver and pancreas in 30 per cent of patients.

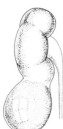
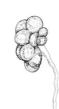
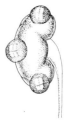

Solitary cyst   Multicystic dysplastic   Multicystic

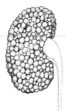
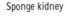

Polycystic   Sponge kidney

Fig. 2.5 Renal cysts.

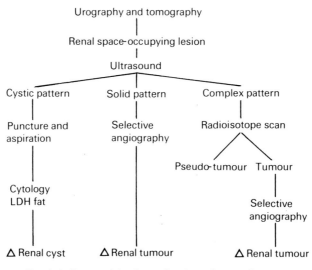

Fig. 2.6 Protocol for investigation of a renal mass.

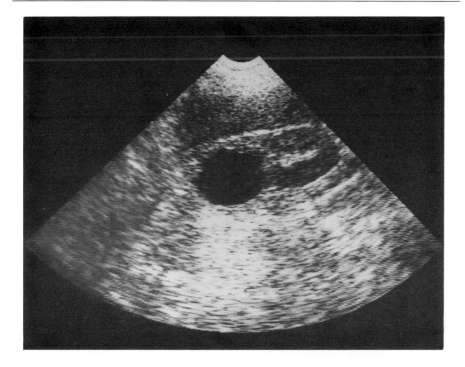

Cyst in Upper Pole of Right Kidney

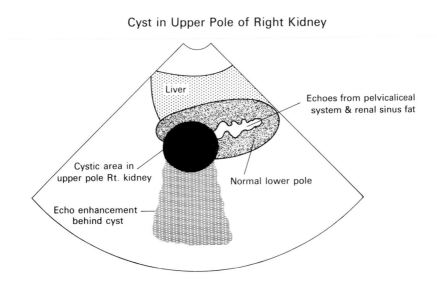

Fig. 2.7 Longitudinal ultrasound scan of a renal cyst in upper pole of right kidney.

Aetiology
Theoretical concept—during renal development imperfect union occurs between the nephrons and collecting tubules. Each kidney contains a million nephrons and potentially a similar number of cysts may develop.

Presentation
Polycystic renal disease presents at two periods in life:

    Infantile variety during the first 9 months.

    Adult variety between 25 and 50 years of age.

    Infantile variety: Gross abdominal distension due to renal masses.

                May cause difficulty with parturition.

                Pale, fretful child with easily palpable kidneys.

  Adult variety: Discovery of renal enlargement on routine abdominal examination.

                Hypertension at insurance examination.

                Haematuria and lethargy with large palpable kidneys.

Investigation
1.   Haemoglobin estimation—anaemia. .
2.   Blood urea estimation—often grossly elevated.
3.   Ultrasound scan—bilateral, lobulated enlargement of both kidneys with echo-free areas within the renal contour.
4.   Selective angiography confirms the presence of multiple renal cysts (*Fig.* 2.8).

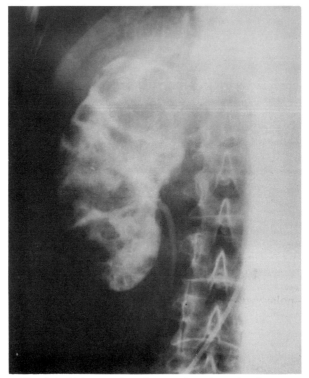

Fig. 2.8 Right renal angiogram in polycystic disease.

5.   IVU—often unrewarding, but may show 'spidery' elongation of renal calices.
6.   Percutaneous renal biopsy—histology confirms polycystic disease.
Treatment
1.   No effective treatment for the primary condition.
2.   Blood transfusions for anaemia: antibiotics for infection.
3.   Chronic renal failure—dialysis and eventual renal transplantation with removal of one or both of the diseased kidneys.
Prognosis
Infantile polycystic cases have a hopeless prognosis and most die before the age of 18 months. Adult polycystic patients may have a normal life span, but may require treatment for renal failure by the age of 55 years (10 per cent of renal transplantation operations are for polycystic disease).
Genetics
Infantile polycystic disease—Mendelian recessive.
Adult polycystic disease—Mendelian dominant—the abnormal gene has a high degree of penetration, but its effects are only apparent in late adult life.

Medullary Sponge Kidney
        Multiple cystic spaces appear in the kidneys at the apex of the renal pyramid, affecting the whole of both kidneys or part of one or both kidneys. The condition presents with recurrent urinary tract infection, and treatment is medical with antibiotics. A medullary sponge kidney has to be distinguished from chronic pyelonephritis and tuberculosis.

•   **B. Renal Trauma**
        Renal injuries may be:
                Direct: Stab wounds, high velocity missiles—associated injuries to liver, spleen, intestine and aorta.
                Indirect: Crush injuries, road traffic accidents, sporting injuries— associated fractures of 11th and 12th ribs and lacerations of liver and spleen.

Pathology
        Degree of renal damage varies from a contusion to avulsion of the renal pedicle (*Fig.* 2.9).
1.   Renal capsule contains bleeding from a cortical tear.
2.   Haematuria results from involvement of renal calix or pelvis.
3.   A cortical tear may extend across the upper or lower pole of the kidney—polar avulsion.
4.   Avulsion of renal pedicle or renal disintegration—severe blood loss.
5.   Delayed rupture—primary bleeding contained by renal capsule bursts through into the perirenal tissues 2–5 days after injury.

Diagnosis
1.   History of trauma, haematuria, hypotension.

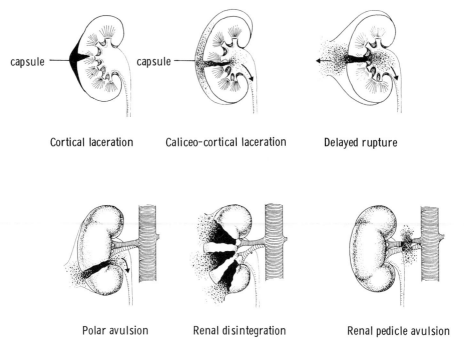

Cortical laceration   Caliceo-cortical laceration   Delayed rupture

Polar avulsion   Renal disintegration   Renal pedicle avulsion

Fig. 2.9 Pathology of renal trauma.

2.   Posterior bruising over lower ribs.
3.   Bimanual examination for a renal mass: often difficult to palpate, due to guarding.
4.   Anterior percussion may demonstrate dullness due to perirenal swelling.
5.   Needle aspiration—may reveal blood in a loin swelling.
6.   Plain X-ray—fractures of 10th, 11th or 12th ribs.
7.   IVU (emergency):
      Often no secretion from injured kidney.
      Demonstrates presence of contralateral kidney.
8.   Cystoscopy—blood efflux from ureteric orifice.
9.   Retrograde ureterography—leakage of dye from renal pelvis into perinephric space (*Fig.* 2.10).

Management
1.   Urgent blood grouping and blood transfusion.
2.   Hourly monitoring of pulse rate and blood pressure.
3.   Collection of all samples of urine for inspection and clinical assessment of the progress of bleeding.
4.   Conservative management in 80 per cent of patients.
5.   20 per cent of patients will require operative treatment.

Surgical Treatment
    Surgical treatment is a life-saving measure in those patients who show a minimal response to intensive resuscitation. Associated liver and splenic injuries

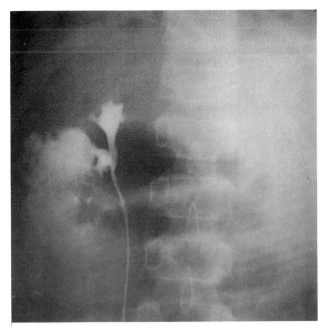

Fig. 2.10 Retrograde ureterography—leakage of contrast from caliceo-cortical rupture of the right kidney.

with intra-abdominal bleeding may force the surgeon to advise surgical exploration (anterior approach). Conservation of functioning renal tissue is the surgical aim in kidney injuries. In the rare injury of pedicle avulsion or renal disintegration a nephrectomy is the only possible operation. Cortical tears and polar lesions are treated by partial nephrectomy.

Sequelae of Renal Trauma

Following trauma, the kidney may show areas of atrophy, cyst or stone formation or chronic pyelonephritis. These sequelae may require surgical treatment months or years after injury to the kidney.

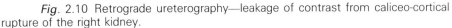

● **C. Infective Disease of the Kidney**
The kidneys may be the site of acute or chronic infection.

Acute Pyelonephritis

Aetiology
Secondary involvement of the renal parenchyma from a blood-borne infection (bacteraemia). 'Acute pyelitis' is not an accurate description of such an infection.

Pathology
The organisms in the renal parenchyma set up micro-inflammatory foci which regress rapidly on treatment. In some instances the foci persist and heal by fibrosis. Repeated acute infection may lead to chronic pyelonephritis.

Symptomatology
1.   Acute onset.
2.   High pyrexia, rigors, sweating.
3.   Dull ache in both loins.
4.   Frequency of micturition, dysuria and micro- or macroscopic haematuria.

Investigations
1.   Turbid urine containing protein and blood on ward testing.
2.   Laboratory examination of urine—organisms, red cells, pus cells and epithelial debris.
3.   Blood culture may isolate organisms.
4.   MSU for culture of organisms and sensitivity to antibiotics.

Treatment
Bed rest, oral fluids, broad spectrum antibiotic therapy (cephaloridine).
Note:
> The healthy kidney is well able to withstand an episode of acute pyelonephritis. Renal function in an obstructed kidney is rapidly compromised in acute infection. Acute pyelonephritis may be the presenting event which leads to the discovery of an obstructive uropathy or chronic pyelonephritis.

Chronic Pyelonephritis

Incidence
The commonest disease of the kidneys, chronic pyelonephritis accounts for 5–9 per cent of all deaths at autopsy. In the United Kingdom 30–35 new cases per million population present for treatment each year.

Aetiology
An insidious disease of unknown aetiology. A systemic auto-immune background has been suggested as a possible aetiological factor.

Pathology
Chronic infection of the renal parenchyma may be caused by non-specific or specific (tuberculous) organisms. Chronic pyelonephritis may present without a previous history of acute infection, though an acute episode frequently draws the clinician's attention to the underlying chronic pathology. One kidney or part of one or both kidneys may be involved. The disease affects both kidneys in the majority of patients. The essential feature is areas of focal fibrosis in the renal

parenchyma—the end result of healing of small cortical abscesses. Contraction and multiplication of the fibrotic lesions lead to destruction of nephrons and chronic renal failure with a contracted kidney. A contracted kidney is small and has an irregular outline, the cortical indentations overlying the 'clubbed' calices (*Fig.* 2.11). Stones may form in the kidney and partial ischaemia of the renal parenchyma with renin release may produce secondary hypertension. Similar changes are sometimes evident in patients suffering from gout and in established vesico-ureteric reflux.

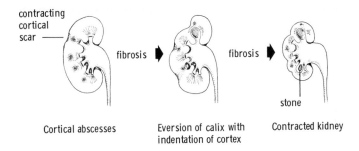

contracting cortical scar

fibrosis ▶   fibrosis ▶

stone

Cortical abscesses   Eversion of calix with   Contracted kidney
                        indentation of cortex

Fig. 2.11 Pathology of chronic pyelonephritis.

Clinical Features
1.   Affects females in child-bearing years.
2.   History of acute infections or recurrent urinary tract infection.
3.   Presenting symptoms:
     Anorexia, headaches, tiredness, aching limbs, thirst, weight loss and haematuria.
4.   Examination:
     Sallow complexion (anaemia), dirty furred tongue with mawkish odour (uraemia), secondary hypertension (one-third of patients).
     The kidneys are never palpable.

Diagnosis
1.   Urine—proteinuria, blood.
2.   Centrifugal deposit:
     White cells in clumps. The urinary white cell examination test estimates the extent of excretion of these cells in urine 3 hr after injection with a bacterial stimulant or a steroid. If the kidney is infected, the white cell excretion rate is doubled in the first hour after injection.
3.   Haematology and biochemistry:
     Low haemoglobin—secondary anaemia.
     ESR—elevated.
     Blood urea—elevated—uraemia.
     Serum creatinine—elevated—uraemia.
4.   DMSA isotope and CT scan. Small kidneys (*Fig.* 1.10).

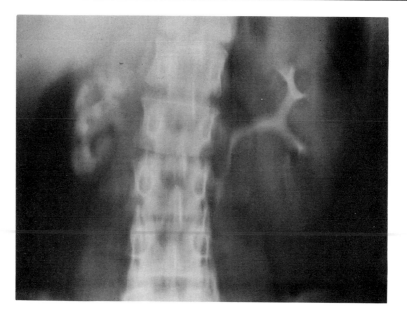

Fig. 2.12 IVU—tomogram showing small scarred right kidney.

5.   IVU. Small kidneys with irregular outline and clubbed calices (*Fig.* 2.12).
6.   Renal biopsy (percutaneous). Histological confirmation of chronic pathology.

Treatment

Chronic pyelonephritis is a progressive disease and arrest of this progression with conservation of renal function must be the primary aim in treatment. Treatment is medical with long-term chemotherapy. Surgical intervention may be indicated for obstruction or ureteric reflux and nephrectomy in the rare event of hypertension resulting from chronic pyelonephritis confined to one kidney. Renal dialysis and renal transplantation are the only hope for advanced cases (60 per cent of patients in a transplant unit have chronic pyelonephritis).

Prognosis

Course of the disease is unpredictable and may be accelerated by recurrent acute infections or may undergo spontaneous remission. Most cases starting in childhood and early adulthood progress to renal failure by middle age. With the advent of renal dialysis and transplantation prognosis for the patient has dramatically improved.

Renal Carbuncle: Perinephric Abscess

A renal carbuncle occurs as the result of secondary metastatic blood-stream infection (*Bacillus, Staphylococcus*) of the renal parenchyma. The primary focus of infection is often a boil, abscess or infected wound. Renal pyaemic

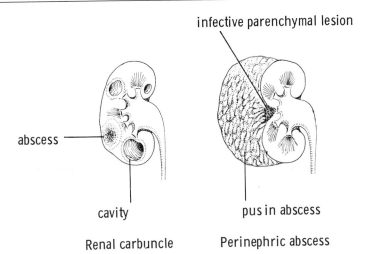

infective parenchymal lesion

abscess

cavity

pus in abscess

Renal carbuncle   Perinephric abscess

Fig. 2.13 Pathology of renal carbuncle and perinephric abscess.

abscesses coalesce to form areas of segmental infection which may perforate the renal capsule and produce a perinephric abscess (*Fig.* 2.13). A perinephric abscess may also arise directly from blood-borne infection of the perinephric space or by direct extension of infection from neighbouring organs, e.g. the colon. The forming abscess will disrupt the renal fascia and may 'point' in the affected loin.

Clinical Features
Severe loin pain, rigors, high swinging pyrexia and a very tender palpable renal mass with overlying pitting oedema of the skin.

Investigations
1.   White cell count grossly elevated with polymorphonuclear leucocytosis.
2.   Blood culture—positive.
3.   Plain abdominal X-ray—loin mass, elevation of diaphragm, medial displacement of gas-filled colon.
4.   Ultrasonography—fluid (blood, pus or urine) around the kidney appears as a transonic area with medial or caudal displacement of kidney.

Treatment
Immediate surgical drainage combined with systemic antibiotic therapy. Co-existing renal pathology is treated later after resolution of the perinephric infection.

● D. Tuberculosis of the Genito-urinary System
Tuberculosis may present as a focal lesion in one part of the genito-urinary tract, but more commonly the whole system is involved in the disease. Tuberculosis is on the wane in Western society but is still prevalent amongst Asian and Far Eastern immigrants to this country.

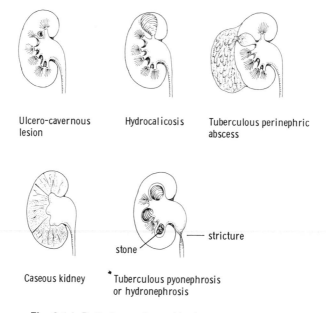

Ulcero-cavernous lesion

Hydrocalicosis

Tuberculous perinephric abscess

Caseous kidney

stone

Tuberculous pyonephrosis or hydronephrosis

stricture

Fig. 2.14 Pathology of renal lesions in tuberculosis.

Pathology (*Fig.* 2.14)

The primary tuberculous focus is in the lung, cervical lymph nodes, intestine or bone, and blood-borne bacilli reach the kidney and are excreted in the urine (tuberculous bacilluria—evident in 21 per cent of patients with pulmonary or skeletal tuberculosis). Only 50 per cent of patients with genito-urinary tuberculosis will have a history of, or evidence of, extra-urogenital infection. Tubercle bacilli in the circulation lodge in glomeruli and form minute tubercles which heal by fibrosis and calcification. In progressive disease several tubercles coalesce to form a cavity (caseation) in the renal papilla which discharges its contents into the renal pelvis (ulcerocavernous lesion) or rarely through the cortex (tuberculous perinephric abscess). Coalescence of a number of caseating cavities destroys the kidney and subsequent calcification results in tuberculous autonephrectomy (*Fig.* 2.15). Caseating material infects the ureteric urothelium, which in turn produces rigidity and thickening of the muscle, fibrosis and stricture formation. Similar infection in the bladder results in a contracted bladder—the ureteric orifices are held rigidly open by the fibrosis—golf-hole ureters. The genital lesions of tuberculosis occur in the epididymis, vas, seminal vesicle and prostate and are either blood-borne or due to direct spread. Urinary and genital tuberculous lesions co-exist in 50 per cent of patients. Tuberculosis of the prostate involves the seminal vesicle and vas (beaded) by retrograde spread. Epididymal tuberculosis is blood-borne; involvement of the scrotal skin forms a cold abscess which may discharge and produce multiple scrotal sinuses. Genito-urinary tuberculosis heals by fibrosis and contraction producing in sequence the following pathology and strictures (*Fig.* 2.16):

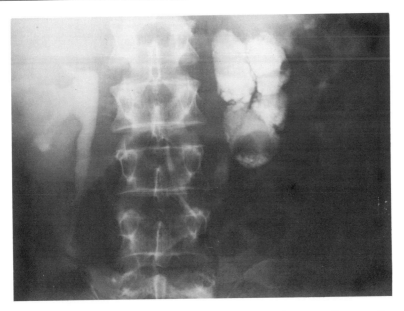

Fig. 2.15 Autonephrectomy of left kidney in long-standing genito-urinary tuberculosis.

1.   Hydrocalicosis.
2.   Pelviureteric stricture.
3.   Hydronephrosis (tuberculous pyonephrosis).
4.   Hydroureter and ureteric stricture.
5.   Contracted bladder.
6.   Urethral stricture (rare).
7.   'Beading' of vas deferens.
8.   Hard 'craggy' enlargement of epididymis—tuberculous epididymitis.
     These pathological changes are often accelerated by the chemotherapeutic drugs used for treatment of tuberculosis.

Clinical Features
1.   Age of presentation—20–40 years.
2.   Haematuria and frequency of micturition.
3.   Febrile illness, weight loss, pallor and night sweats.
4.   Adult male may present with tuberculous epididymitis (25 per cent).
5.   Advanced cases—cachexia, gross frequency of micturition, multiple scrotal sinuses and palpable kidneys.

Note:
     In most patients there will be a positive history of familial tuberculosis.

Diagnosis
1.   The Mantoux test will be positive.
2.   Ward examination of urine—protein and red blood cells.
3.   Microscopical examination of urine—pus cells but no organisms—sterile pyuria.

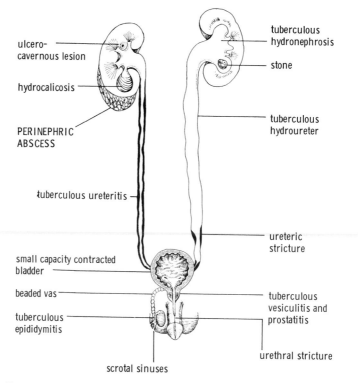

ulcero-cavernous lesion

hydrocalicosis

PERINEPHRIC ABSCESS

tuberculous ureteritis

small capacity contracted bladder

beaded vas

tuberculous epididymitis

scrotal sinuses

tuberculous hydronephrosis

stone

tuberculous hydroureter

ureteric stricture

tuberculous vesiculitis and prostatitis

urethral stricture

Fig. 2.16 Pathological complications of genito-urinary tuberculosis.

4. Three early morning specimens—stained by Ziehl-Neelsen—isolation of TB.
5. Urine culture—Lowenstein's media—growth of TB—sensitivity ascertained.
6. ESR—persistently elevated.
7. Guinea-pig inoculation of urine—growth of TB in vivo after 6 weeks.
8. IVU—calcification in renal cortex, hydrocalicosis, pelvi-ureteric and ureteric strictures, hydroureter and hydronephrosis, caseous kidney and autonephrectomy (non-functioning), contracted bladder.
9. Endoscopy—tubercles around ureteric orifices, golf-hole ureters, contracted small capacity bladder (maximum capacity not greater than 80 ml of fluid).

Treatment

Medical Treatment
1. Antituberculous drugs, depending on sensitivity of TB organisms.
2. Drugs alternated to combat resistance.
3. Treatment for 18–24 months.
4. 5-year survival and cure rate is 90 per cent.

Surgical Treatment
1. Necessary in 5–10 per cent of patients.
2. Surgery for obstructive uropathy.
3. Enlarging bladder capacity.
4. Undertaken under full antituberculosis therapy cover.

Operations
1. Nephroureterectomy—removal of caseous kidney or TB pyonephrosis in continuity with the ureter (*Fig.* 2.29).
2. Partial nephrectomy—excision of part of kidney for localized TB: hydrocalicosis and stone formation (*Fig.* 2.28).
3. Cavernostomy—drainage of a tuberculous abscess in kidney.
4. Ureteric strictures
   Upper end—reimplantation into renal pelvis.
   Lower end—reimplantation into bladder,
   Multiple—ureteric replacement—neoureteroplasty (*Fig.* 4.8).
5. Ileo- or colocystoplasty: enlargement of bladder capacity by isolated vascularized loop of ileum or colon (*Fig.* 5.23).
6. Urinary diversion—in advanced cases with obstructive uropathy and impending chronic renal failure.
7. Epididymectomy—removal of diseased epididymis and scrotal sinuses not responding to antituberculous therapy.

● **E. Renal Tumours**
Tumours of the kidney account for 2 per cent of all malignancies and are benign or malignant.

Classification and Incidence
Benign—haemangioma, hamartoma, fibroma, adenoma, lipoma.
Malignant:
   Congenital—Nephroblastoma (Wilms)—10 per cent
   Acquired:
      Parenchymal:
         Carcinoma   78 per cent
         Fibrosarcoma ⎱ 2 per cent
         Liposarcoma ⎰
      Renal pelvis:
         Transitional cell ⎱ 10 per cent
         Squamous cell   ⎰
Benign tumours of the kidney are very rare. A haemangioma produces profuse haematuria with clot colic and mimics tumours of the renal pelvis.

Nephroblastoma (Wilms' Tumour)

Incidence
1.   Tumour of infancy and childhood: peak incidence 2 years.
2.   Equal sex distribution.
3.   Bilateral in 5 per cent.
4.   Commonest genito-urinary neoplasm in infancy.
5.   Second to brain tumours as cause of death in this age group.
6.   Has been recorded in adults.

Aetiology
Unknown: may be explained by an embryological metaplasia.

Pathology
1.   Rapidly growing parenchymal tumour producing compression of the renal cortex and distortion of the calices as it expands.
2.   Transected tumour is well encapsulated and greyish-white in appearance with cystic spaces, haemorrhage and areas of papillary growth.
3.   Histology:
         Undifferentiated embryonic tumour with primitive glomeruli and tubules and containing irregular areas of collagenous, cartilagenous, osseous and adipose tissue.
4.   Rarely secretes renin—hypertension.

Spread of Tumour (*Fig.* 2.17)

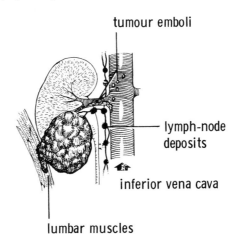

Fig. 2.17 Dissemination of nephroblastoma and renal carcinoma. Note direct growth of tumour within lumen of renal vein.

1.   Local infiltration:
         Lumbar muscles, colon, duodenum, pancreas, and anterior abdominal wall.

2.   Lymphatic:
            Renal vein nodes, pancreatic, mediastinal and distant nodes.
3.   Blood stream:
            Tumour emboli or direct spread inside renal veins into vena cava,
            liver, lungs, long bones and brain.

Tumour Staging
As for renal carcinoma (p. 43).

Clinical Features
1.   Visible abdominal mass in a thin infant, with pallor, lassitude and anorexia.
2.   One-third of patients will have haematuria.
3.   In 10 per cent of patients distant metastases are the presenting feature.

Examination
1.   Palpable mass in upper abdomen and flank.
2.   Abdominal distension with prominent veins indicates ascites and caval
        obstruction.
3.   Lymphadenopathy—distant lymph node metastases.
4.   Hepatomegaly—liver secondary deposits.
5.   Physical signs in the chest, indicating pulomary metastases.

Investigations
1.   Urine examined—red blood cells.
2.   Blood picture—secondary anaemia.
3.   Chest X-ray—pulmonary metastases or pleural effusion.
4.   Ultrasound—renal mass: differentiation between a solid and cystic lesion
        (see protocol on p. 26), liver enlargement.
5.   IVU—parenchymal mass, caliceal distortion and compression, areas of
        speckled calcification (*Fig.* 2.18).
6.   Vena cavography—involvement of renal vein and vena cava.

Differential Diagnosis
1.   Neuroblastoma—adrenal tumour—displaces the kidney caudally.
2.   Hydronephrosis—diagnosed by ultrasound.

Treatment
1.   In all cases radical nephrectomy (*Fig.* 2.27) with early ligation of renal vein.
2.   In all cases postoperative combination chemotherapy—actinomycin D,
        vinblastine and adriamycin.
3.   In fixed tumours—radiotherapy to renal area.

Prognosis
1.   T1 and T2 tumours with no local spread or distant metastases—80 per cent
        5-year survival.
2.   T3, N1 and N2 tumours with no distant metastases—30 per cent 5-year
        survival.
3.   T4, N3 or 4, M1 tumours—none survive 5 years.

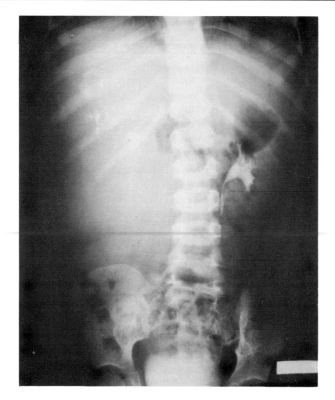

Fig. 2.18 IVU distortion of the calices and calcification in a nephroblastoma of the right kidney.

Adenocarcinoma of the Kidney (Hypernephroma; Grawitz Tumour; Clear-cell Carcinoma)

A carcinoma arising from the renal tubules.

Incidence
1. Commoner in males than females (3 to 2 incidence male : female).
2. Usually present after 40 years of age.
3. Accounts for 2 per cent of all male malignant tumours.

Pathology
1. Well-encapsulated, lobulated tumour, golden yellow in colour, radiating septa and areas of haemorrhage or necrosis.
2. Histology—sheets of columnar or cuboidal cells with clear cytoplasm and small dark nuclei. Cytoplasmic fat and cholesterol produce yellow colour.

Spread of Tumour (*Fig*. 2.17).
1. Direct infiltration—lumbar muscles and diaphragm, colon, duodenum.
2. Lymphatic—nodes along renal vein, para-aortic, mediastinal and distant nodes.

3. Blood stream—bones (ribs and vertebrae), lungs and liver.
4. In 40 per cent of patients the renal vein and vena cava are involved.

Associated Changes
1. Elevated ESR—changes in serum proteins—50 per cent of patients.
2. Hypertension—renin secretion by tumour—30 per cent of patients.
3. Anaemia—depression of erythropoiesis—30 per cent of patients.
4. Weight loss—depression of appetite by tumour metastases—30 per cent of patients.
5. Pyrexia—circulating pyrogens—20 per cent of patients.
6. Elevated alkaline phosphatase—tumour secretion—10 per cent of patients.
7. Hypercalcaemia—tumour secretion of parathormone—5 per cent of patients.
8. Polycythaemia—secretion of erythropoietin—4 per cent of patients.

Tumour Staging
International TNM classification. Staging depends on results of preoperative investigations, operative findings and pathological examination of the excised specimens.

> T1—small tumour without enlargement of the kidney.
> T2—large tumour without extrarenal spread.
> T3—spread of tumour into perinephric fat.
> T4—extension into neighbouring organs: fixation to the abdominal wall.
> N0—no regional node involvement.
> N1—single regional node involved.
> N2—multiple regional nodes involved.
> N3—fixed regional node involvement.
> N4—involvement of distant nodes in the body.
> M0—no metastases.
> M1—distant metastases.

Clinical Features
1. Triad of symptoms—pain in the loin, haematuria and tumour.
2. Haematuria—tumour invasion of calix—clot colic, 'tea-leaf' clots in urine—60 per cent.
3. Discovery of tumour—by patient or clinician—20 per cent.
4. Distant metastases—haemoptysis, pathological fractures, lower limb oedema due to caval obstruction—10 per cent.
5. Anaemia and elevated ESR—'silent' renal tumour—10 per cent.
6. Rare presentation—polycythaemia, hypertension, pyrexia of unknown origin, hypercalcaemia.

Investigations and Diagnosis
The protocol for investigation of a renal mass is described on p. 26 (*Fig.* 2.6).
1. Urine—red blood cells.
2. Blood—haemoglobin estimation—for anaemia and polycythaemia.
3. ESR—non-specific elevation in 50 per cent of patients.

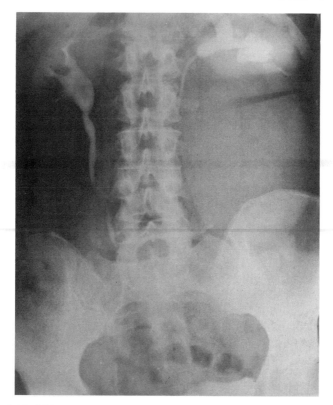

Fig. 2.19 IVU—compression and displacement of the renal pelvis and calices by a large carcinoma of the lower pole of the left kidney.

4.   Chest X-ray—pulmonary metastases, pleural effusion.
5.   IVU and tomography—delineation of mass: displacement and distortion of calices (*Fig.* 2.19).
6.   Ultrasonography—differentiation between tumour and cyst of kidney or hydronephrosis. Dense echoes from tumour (*Fig.* 2.20).
7.   Selective renal angiography—renal arterial pattern: vascular blush in tumour is diagnostic (*Fig.* 2.21).
8.   Vena cavography—invasion of renal vein: erase obstruction of vena cava.

Treatment
In all cases radical nephrectomy (*Fig.* 2.27) where possible.
1.   T1 and T2 tumours—anterior or thoraco-abdominal approach with early ligation of renal vein.
2.   T3 and T4 tumours—invasion of perinephric fat, local fixation, lymph node involvement, renal vein involvement—nephrectomy and radiotherapy.
3.   Chemotherapy has not proved effective in treatment.
4.   Selective tumour embolization under radiological control (p. 18) for

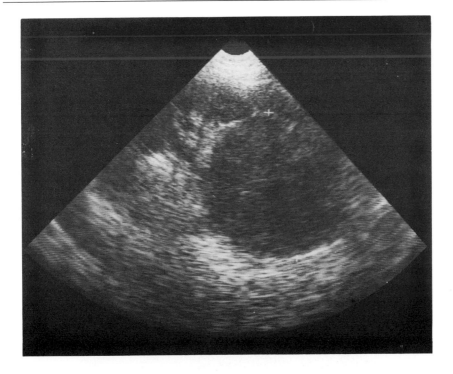

Renal Cell Carcinoma of Left Kidney

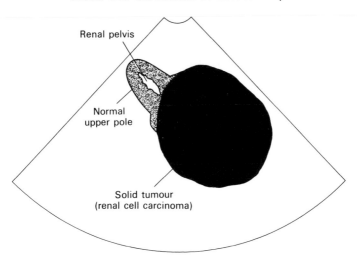

Fig. 2.20 Ultrasound scan showing dense echoes from a renal tumour.

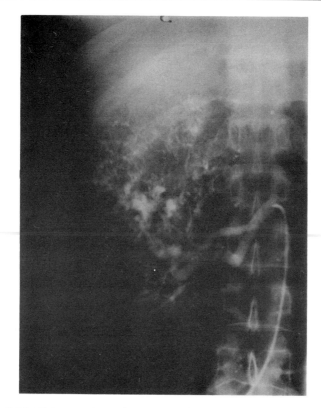

Fig. 2.21 Right renal angiogram—pathological circulation in a renal cell carcinoma.

palliative treatment of elderly or critically ill patients with an adenocarcinoma of the kidney.

Prognosis
The 5-year survival rate for well-differentiated adenocarcinoma of the kidney (T1 and T2 tumours) is 40 per cent.

Carcinoma of the Renal Pelvis

Incidence
10 per cent of all renal tumours.
Bilateral in 25 per cent of patients.

Aetiology
Similar aetiological features to those producing urothelial bladder tumours (p. 107).
May be associated with analgesic drug abuse.

Pathology
There are two types of histology:
1. Transitional cell carcinoma—single or multiple tumours of the urothelium in the renal pelvis (90 per cent).
2. Squamous cell carcinoma—(very rare: 10 per cent)—arising from metaplastic changes in urothelium of the pelvis due to irritation from a renal calculus.

Symptomatology
Loin pain, profuse haematuria and clot colic (spindle-shaped clots).

Diagnosis
1. Urine cytology—malignant cells in urine.
2. IVU—filling defect in the renal pelvis (*Fig.* 2.22).
3. Diagnostic retrograde urography—filling defect in renal pelvis.

Treatment
Nephroureterectomy with excision of a cuff of bladder urothelium around the ureteric orifice (*Fig.* 2.29).

Prognosis
Excellent. Prompt diagnosis due to early onset of haematuria. Squamous cell carcinoma of the renal pelvis has a poor prognosis.
Note:
In 25 per cent of cases the tumours are bilateral.
Prolonged follow-up examination of the bladder and the remaining kidney are essential in order to exclude the development of further urothelial tumours.

● **F. Renal Vascular Disorders: Hypertension**
Goldblatt's animal experiments demonstrated that partial renal ischaemia released renin and produced hypertension. In man, the vascular lesions which affect renal function and may contribute to development of secondary hypertension are summarized in *Fig.* 2.23.

Aetiology
1. Young patients under 45 years of age—hypertension—fibromuscular hyperplasia of the wall of the renal artery—renal artery stenosis.
2. Older patients—hypertension—atheromatous changes at junction of renal artery with aorta—partial renal ischaemia.

Note:
The elderly patient may have generalized atheromatous changes in all central and peripheral arteries.

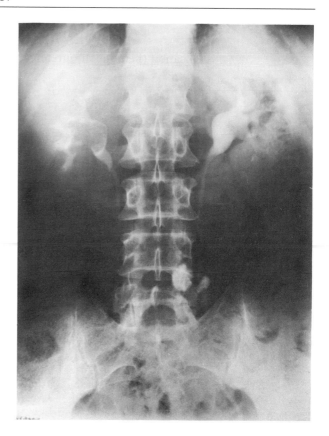

Diagnosis

Young hypertensive, under 45 years of age—a vascular bruit may be heard over the aorta and stenosed renal artery.

IVU—excretion and clearance of dye in the affected side is delayed for some 10 min as compared with the normal contralateral kidney.

Selective renal angiography and digital vascular imaging demonstrate the narrowed segment of artery (*Fig.* 2.24).

Treatment

Transluminal angioplasty—dilatation and stretching of the stenosis during selective angiography—is the method of choice for the management of the renal artery stenosis. The surgical procedures used for the relief of ischaemia from stenosis or atheroma of the renal artery are shown in *Fig.* 2.25.

Prognosis

1. Stenotic group—60 per cent success after reconstructive surgery.
2. Atheromatous group—disappointing results after reconstructive surgery.

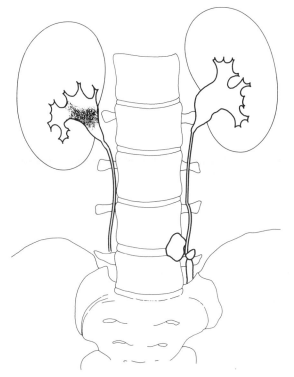

Fig. 2.22 IVU—urothelial tumour of right renal pelvis.

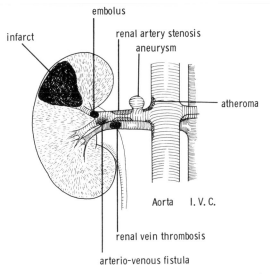

Fig. 2.23 Pathology of renal ischaemia and hypertension.

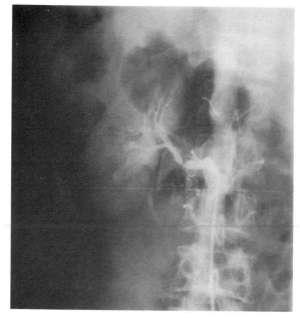

Fig. 2.24 Selective angiography—renal artery stenosis.

Future Developments

Autotransplantation
Removal of the kidney from the loin, excision of the stenotic segment (bench surgery) and replacement of the kidney into the iliac fossa on the same side.

Other Arterial Lesions
1.   Embolism:
           Subacute bacterial endocarditis—parenchymal infarct—partial or total nephrectomy.
2.   Thrombosis:
           Occlusion of renal artery distal to obstruction by atheroma or stenosis—nephrectomy.
3.   Aneurysm:
           Congenital or traumatic—nephrectomy or autotransplantation and bench surgery.
4.   Arteriovenous fistula:
           Trauma from penetrating wound or renal surgery—loud bruit.
           Nephrectomy or autotransplantation and bench surgery.
5.   Renal vein thrombosis:
           Exclusively affects neonates and infants.
           Complication of fulminating systemic infection.
           Treatment
                Nephrectomy if unilateral.
                Bilateral renal vein thrombosis is universally fatal.

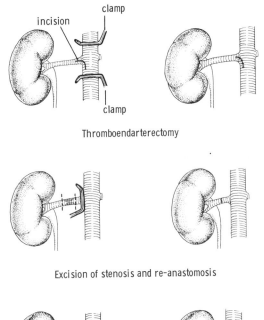

Thromboendarterectomy

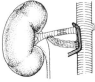

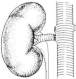

Excision of stenosis and re-anastomosis

By-pass Teflon graft   Re-implantation of renal artery

Fig. 2.25 Reconstructive procedures for the treatment of renal artery stenosis and atheroma.

● **G. Nephrectomy**

Surgical Approaches to the Kidney
1. Posterior lumbar with or without resection of 12th rib—standard approach.
2. Anterior transperitoneal or extraperitoneal—for exposure of renal vessels.
3. Lateral thoraco-abdominal—reserved for radical nephrectomy for a maligant tumour or large renal mass.
    There are four types of nephrectomy—total, radical, partial and nephroureterectomy.
1. Total nephrectomy (*Fig.* 2.26).

kidney in perinephric fat

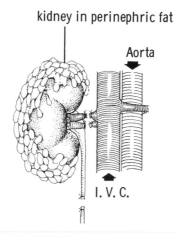

Fig. 2.26 Total nephrectomy.

Indication—congenital anomalies, traumatized kidneys, chronic infection (pyelonephritis), obstructive uropathy, large staghorn calculi, ischaemic kidneys, and palliative removal of a malignant tumour.

2. Radical nephrectomy (*Fig.* 2.27).
    Indication—malignant renal tumours.
3. Partial nephrectomy (*Fig.* 2.28).
    Indication—renal laceration, segmental infection in chronic pyelonephritis or tuberculosis, calculous disease of upper or lower calix, benign renal tumours and rarely for a malignant tumour in a solitary kidney.
4. Nephroureterectomy (*Fig.* 2.29).

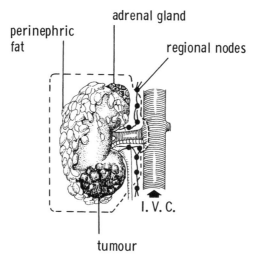

Fig. 2.27 Radical nephrectomy.

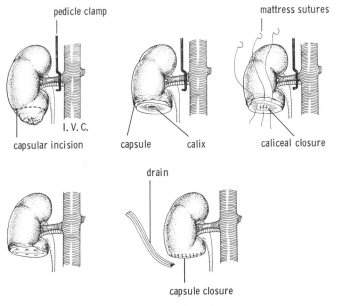

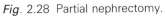

Fig. 2.28 Partial nephrectomy.

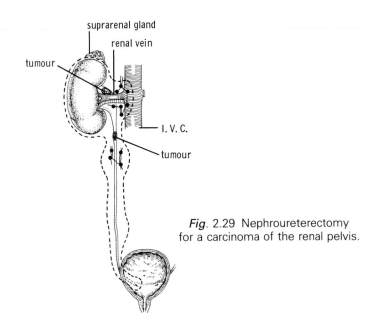

Fig. 2.29 Nephroureterectomy
for a carcinoma of the renal pelvis.

Indication—duplex kidneys with pyelonephritis of one half of the renal duplication (hemi-nephroureterectomy), renal tuberculosis, carcinoma of the renal pelvis.

Complications of Nephrectomy

1.   Haemorrhage:

Primary—at time of operation from renal pedicle.

Secondary—24 hr or more after renal operation.

2.   Infection:

Subphrenic abscess.

Wound infection in first week after operation.

Delayed infection from bed of kidney—discharging sinuses in operation scar.

3

Urolithiasis

In theory, calculi could form in the urinary tract wherever urine and its contained solutes are in contact with the urothelium. In practice, stones form in the kidney and the bladder. Ureteric calculi are in transit from the kidney to the bladder. There are two types of urinary calculi:

1. Primary:
   Develop in a normal urinary tract, in acid urine and in metabolic disease.
2. Secondary:
   Develop in infected alkaline urine and in obstructive uropathy.

- **A. Renal Calculi**
  The aetiology of renal calculi is unknown.

Suggested Theory of Renal Stone Formation

Primary calculi form in the suburothelial plane of a renal papilla, resulting in erosion of papilla, precipitation of urinary crystalloids on the nidus, and stone formation.

Secondary calculi result from bacteria, debris and inflammatory products in infected and alkaline urine precipitating within the renal tract and forming a stone.

There are five varieties of formed calculi (*Fig.* 3.1):

1. Calcium oxalate (80 per cent)—radio-opaque, hard and pale yellow with sharp projections (mulberry calculus)—alkaline urine.

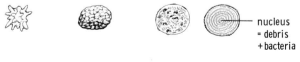

Oxalate stone
(Mulberry stone)   Uric acid stone   Mixed stone

nucleus
= debris
+ bacteria

Fig. 3.1 Common types of urinary calculi.

2. Phosphate (10 per cent)—compound of calcium, magnesium and ammonium phosphate (triple phosphate), radio-opaque, chalky white stone, often large (staghorn calculus)—strong alkaline urine.
3. Uric acid (8 per cent)—radio-lucent, faceted and multiple, light brown in colour—acid urine.
4. Cystine (2 per cent)—radio-opaque due to sulphur content: metabolic stone due to excessive tubular excretion of cystine and amino acids—acid urine.
5. Xanthine and pyruvate stones—rare, result of inborn errors of purine metabolism—acid urine.

Predisposing Factors in Renal Urolithiasis

Renal Stones
Renal stones may be either idiopathic, the causes being dietary, dehydration, stasis or infection, or metabolic, due to primary hyperparathyroidism, idiopathic hypercalcaemia, milk–alkali syndrome, hypervitaminosis D, sarcoidosis, multiple myelomatosis, cystinuria, inborn errors of purine metabolism.

●   **B. Bladder Stones**

Incidence and Aetiology
1. Middle East, Far East, Turkey—idiopathic calculi, dietary factors (malnutrition), dehydration (concentration of urinary solutes), infection.
2. Egypt and East Africa—bilharzia—acquired stone.
3. Western society—bladder outflow obstruction, bladder diverticulae, foreign bodies in bladder, post-irradiation, stasis and infection.

●   **C. Ureteric Calculi**
Stones do not form in the ureter, except in the obstructed ureter (megaureter). Small stones pass from renal pelvis to bladder via the ureter.

Formation of Urinary Calculi (*Fig.* 3.2)
Eighty per cent of stones are found in relation to the lower calix of the kidney. A calculus developing in a renal papilla will either remain and enlarge in the renal parenchyma or ulcerate through into the renal pelvis. Within the pelvis the stone may continue to enlarge (silent stone) and in an infected alkaline urine may form a staghorn calculus, associated with chronic inflammation of the pelvic urothelium or, rarely, squamous metaplasia. The majority of calculi leave the renal pelvis and migrate down the ureter. Arrest occurs at three points in the ureter—the pelviureteric junction, at the pelvic bony brim and in the terminal ureter (*Fig.* 1.3) producing stasis, hydroureter and hydronephrosis with

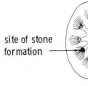
site of stone formation

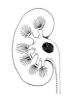

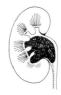

Stone forms at apex of renal papilla

Stone in renal pelvis

Staghorn calculus in renal pelvis

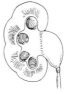

Staghorn calculus

Stone impacted in pelvi-ureteric junction

Fig. 3.2 Renal stone formation.

subsequent development of a ureteric stricture in some instances. Within the bladder the stone may be retained and enlarge or be voided in the urine. Large bladder calculi are often associated with squamous metaplasia of the bladder urothelium. Stone impaction in the urethra is possible but rare, and occurs in its narrowest segment, viz. the terminal 2·5 cm.

Clinical Features

Three cardinal symptoms of urolithiasis are pain, haematuria and dysuria. An impacted stone in the renal parenchyma is painless, causing occasional haematuria and dysuria.

Stone in Renal Pelvis
1. Silent, occasional haematuria and dysuria.
2. Impaction in pelvi-ureteric junction—renal colic.
3. Pain—continuous boring pain in the loin, aggravated by jolting or movement, micro- or macroscopic haematuria.
4. Staghorn calculus and large pelvic calculi—often painless, urine always contains red blood cells, protein, pus cells and epithelial débris.

Stone in Ureter
Ureteric colic—violent colicky pain in loin radiating to groin and genitalia associated with shock and vomiting. Haematuria is frequently present due to damage to the urothelium by the stone.

Bladder Stone
Relatively painless. Terminal haematuria, dysuria and interruption of urine flow

are due to impaction of the stone in the internal urinary meatus during micturition.

Physical Examination

Often unrewarding. Loin tenderness indicates a urinary infection or distension of the renal pelvis due to obstruction. The kidney is rarely palpable. An impacted ureteric calculus will produce shock and vomiting, and the intense pain of ureteric colic. Prostatic enlargement and a clinically palpable and distended bladder may be associated with a bladder stone.

Diagnosis and Investigation

Patients with calculous disease of the urinary tract present in three ways:
1. With renal pain or ureteric colic—urgent.
2. With urinary tract symptoms—pain, haematuria, dysuria—semi-urgent.
3. Incidental discovery of urolithiasis on abdominal X-rays for other reasons—non-urgent.

Urgent Investigation for Renal Pain or Ureteric Colic

1. Urine examination for red blood cells, protein and infective organisms. Plain X-ray of abdomen (*Fig.* 3.3)—70 per cent of calculi are radio-opaque.

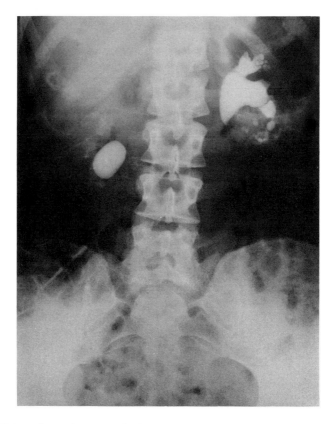

Fig. 3.3 Plain radiograph—stone in right renal pelvis and a left staghorn calculus.

2.   IVU (emergency) for size and site of impaction of calculus and secondary effects on the upper urinary tract plus functional state of contralateral kidney.
3.   Delayed films are taken 2, 3, 4–12 hr after the injection if the obstructed kidney shows no function in the early stage of excretion.

Routine Investigation for Urinary Tract Symptoms or Incidental Discovery of a Calculus

1.   Specific biochemical and urinary examination for oxalate and other crystalloids.
2.   Urinary amino acid estimation to exclude disorder of purine metabolism.
3.   Serial blood calcium estimations to exclude primary hyperparathyroidism.
4.   Creatinine clearance test for renal function.
5.   Ultrasonography—demonstrates renal enlargement, hydronephrosis and hydroureter: intrapelvic or intraureteric stones appear as high echogenic areas within the dilated urinary tract: bladder stones have high echogenicity in a fluid-filled bladder.
6.   Plain abdominal film—demonstration of calcification or radio-opaque calculi in the urinary tract (*Fig.* 1.7).
7.   IVU and tomography—localization of calculi in the kidney, renal pelvis, ureter and bladder.
8.   Radioisotope renography—estabish differential renal function.
9.   Cystoscopic diagnosis of bladder calculi (number and size) and assessment of bladder outlet and prostate gland.
10.   Retrograde pyelography—establish site of calculous impaction in the ureter.

Management and Treatment of Urolithiasis

Treatment falls into two well-defined categories:
1.   Management of acute symptoms produced by a stone impacted in the pelvi-ureteric junction or passing down the ureter—urgent.
2.   Management of an established stone in the urinary tract—routine.

Management of acute symptoms.
The pain of ureteric colic is severe. Hospital admission, bed rest, oral fluids and liberal i.m. injections of pethidine, morphine and an antispasmodic, e.g. Buscopan. All urine is collected and sieved to retrieve a calculus that may be voided. An emergency IVU may demonstrate site of stone impaction and progress of the stone, if radio-opaque, is monitored by daily plain abdominal films. The acute phase lasts 3–12 hr but the colic may recur at intervals as the stone passes down the ureter. A calculus that is moving towards the bladder and is not producing progressive hydronephrosis is safely left for 6 weeks—its progress down the ureter is recorded by a limited IVU after 3 weeks.

Indications for Early Surgery for a Ureteric Stone

1.   Hydronephrosis with infection behind the stone—urgent removal of stone.
2.   Stone size and shape:
         Rounded stone greater than 4 mm in diameter—operation—ureterolithotomy (*Fig.* 3.4).

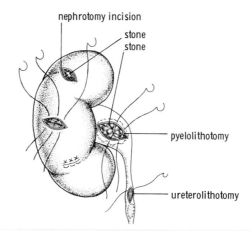

nephrotomy incision

stone

stone

pyelolithotomy

ureterolithotomy

Fig. 3.4 Nephrolithotomy: pyelolithotomy: ureterolithotomy.

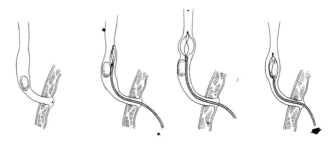

Stone in lower ureter   Dormia catheter in situ   Stone engaged in
                                                           Dormia basket

Fig. 3.5 Dormia stone dislodger.

Spindle-shaped stone less than 4 mm in diameter in the lower ureter—Dormia stone dislodger—successful in 60–70 per cent (*Fig.* 3.5), or removal by retrograde ureteroscopy.

3. Impaction of stone after 6 weeks—formal removal by a dislodger, ureteroscopy or open operation.

Note:

Stricture of the ureter may occur years later after stone impaction or surgery for removal of the stone.

Management of an Established Stone in the Kidney and Renal Pelvis

Surgical aim is to relieve upper tract obstruction and eliminate the possibility of continued infection of the urinary tract. A symptomless or silent stone in the renal pelvis will, over the years, produce deterioration of renal function.

General Principles

1. A symptomless renal or staghorn calculus in an elderly patient is best left alone.

2. A symptomless renal parenchymal stone is removed by nephrolithotomy (*Fig.* 3.4) or partial nephrectomy (*Fig.* 2.28).

3.   A stone in the renal pelvis is removed by pyelolithotomy (*Fig.* 3.4), percutaneous or extracorporeal lithotripsy, nephrolithotomy (*Fig.* 3.4). (*See below*—Recent developments.)
4.   A staghorn calculus in a non-functioning kidney—total nephrectomy (*Fig.* 2.26).
5.   A staghorn calculus with renal function—pyelolithotomy and percutaneous operative nephroscopy or extracorporeal lithotripsy.

Stones in the Bladder
Treatment of bladder stones depends on their size, consistency and number.

A single soft stone up to 4 cm in diameter or multiple small stones can be crushed endoscopically (lithalopaxy) and the remnants washed away.

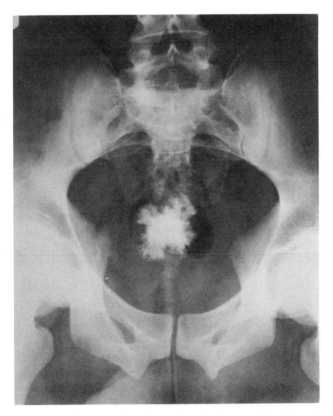

Fig. 3.6 Plain radiograph showing a large spiculated bladder calculus.

Larger stones and hard stones (*Fig.* 3.6)—open operation—suprapubic cystotomy (*Fig.* 5.19).

Bladder stones in association with outlet obstruction are removed at open operation in conjunction with surgery for relief of the obstruction, e.g. prostatectomy.

Recent Developments
Percutaneous Nephrolithotomy
Stones of small size in the renal pelvis and upper ureter are visualized by a percutaneously introduced nephroscope. The stones are extracted by grasping forceps or disintegrated by ultrasound or electrohydraulic waves. Stone remnants are washed away through the nephroscope or pass spontaneously down the ureter.
Extracorporeal Lithotripsy
Disintegration of stones in the renal pelvis is achieved by high frequency ultrasound waves applied externally by a lithotriptor, the patient being immersed in a saline bath. The technique is under investigation in two centres in this country. Facilities must be available for subsequent percutaneous recovery of stone fragments from the renal pelvis.
Operative Retrograde Ureteroscopy
Operative ureteroscopes are available which may allow stone crushing and extraction from the ureter under direct vision, or disintegration of the stone by ultrasound.

Prognosis and Prevention of Urinary Calculi
Recurrent stone formation occurs in 15–20 per cent of patients due to incomplete removal of the stone or failure to deal with coexisting pathology at the time of operation.
Metabolic stones are preventable:
1.   Oxaluria—avoid high oxalate foods, strawberries, rhubarb, tomatoes.
2.   Uric acid stones—alkalinization of urine and allopurinol.
3.   Cystine stones—alkalinization of urine.
4.   Calcium-containing stones—thiazide diuretic: cellulose phosphate.
5.   Hyperparathyroidism—excision of parathyroid adenoma or tumour.
There is no known method of preventing recurrence of the common 'mixed' type of calculus—adequate treatment of urinary tract infection and a high fluid intake may be beneficial.

4

The ureter

● **A. Congenital Anomalies of the Ureter**

Ureteric Duplication

1. Duplication of the ureter is found in 1 per cent of all autopsies.
2. In incomplete duplication both ureters join at a point between the renal pelvis and bladder.
3. In complete duplication both ureters open separately into the bladder, the ureter from the upper part of the kidney opening caudal to the ureter from the lower renal segment (*Fig.* 4.1).
4. In 10 per cent of complete duplications one ureter is ectopic and opens into

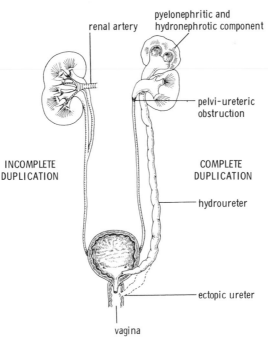

Fig. 4.1 Ureteric duplication.

the urethra or vagina below the bladder neck. The ectopic ureter may have an associated ureterocele which presents in the infant vagina. One or both of the duplicated ureters may have a pelvi-ureteric stenosis or may reflux.
5.   The kidney draining into the duplicated ureters has two components (pyelon duplex). One half of the pyelon is often dysplastic and pyelonephritic with associated hydronephrosis, hydroureter and ureteric reflux.

Clinical Features
1.   Incomplete duplication:
      Symptomless, often a chance finding.
2.   Complete duplication:
      50 per cent symptomless.
      50 per cent dysuria and haematuria due to infection of the dysplastic hemi-pyelon.
      Ectopic ureter—diurnal incontinence—wet by day and night.

Diagnosis
IVU demonstrates the anomaly (*Fig.* 4.2)—absence of a major calix if half the pyelon duplex is non-functioning.

On cystoscopy, two ureteric orifices are visible. The ectopic ureteric opening may be seen in posterior urethra in male or vaginal fornix in female.

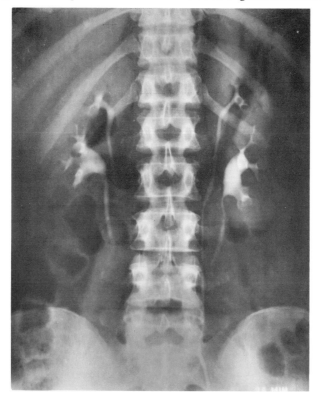

Fig. 4.2 IVU—bilateral complete ureteric duplication.

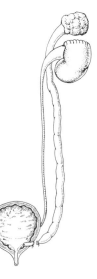

Fig. 4.3 Heminephroureterectomy.

Treatment

Incontinent ectopic ureter—surgical excision—heminephroureterectomy (*Fig.* 4.3). Dysplasia and infection of one half of pyelon duplex with or without ureteric reflux—excision of one half of kidney with its associated ureter—heminephroureterectomy.

Retrocaval Ureter

A rare anomaly. The right ureter runs medially behind the vena cava and crosses the cava anteriorly to enter the bladder on the right side of the trigone. Treatment is not indicated, but the abnormally sited ureter may cause diagnostic difficulties during abdominal operations (*Fig.* 4.4).

Ureterocele

Dilatation of the terminal ureter within the bladder wall associated either with a normally placed ureteric orifice or, rarely, an ectopic orifice (*Fig.* 4.5). Bilateral in 15 per cent of patients. The ureterocele may become very large and may occupy most of the available space in the bladder.

Clinical Features

1. Obstruction to the bladder neck in both sexes.
2. Secondary infection—dysuria and haematuria.
3. Ectopic ureterocele in female—presents as a vaginal tumour at birth.

Diagnosis

IVU typically shows a crescent-moon appearance or a rounded swelling in the cystogram phase (*Fig.* 4.6) with associated hydroureter and vesico-ureteric reflux.

Cystoscopy confirms the diagnosis.

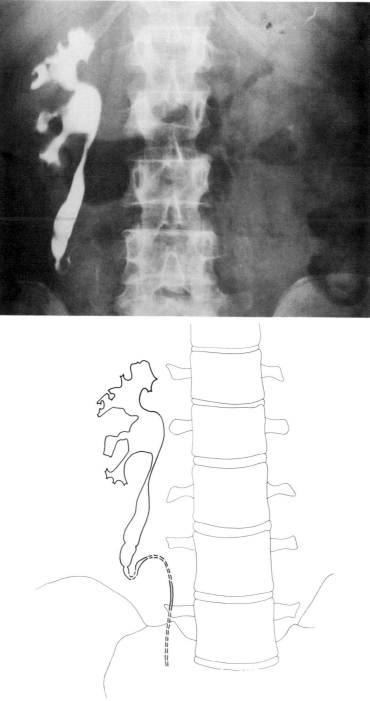

Fig. 4.4 Retrograde ureterogram—retrocaval ureter.

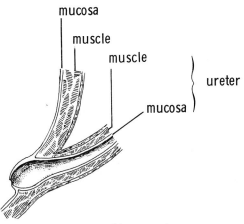

Fig. 4.5 Ureterocele.

Treatment

1. Uncomplicated ureterocele:
   No treatment or endoscopic diathermy excision.
2. Hydroureter and stone formation:
   Transvesical excision and reimplantation of ureter.
3. Ectopic ureterocele:
   Heminephroureterectomy (*Fig.* 4.3).
4. Non-functioning kidney:
   Nephroureterectomy and excision of ureterocele (*Fig.* 2.29).

- ## B. Ureteric Trauma

  Injury to the ureter may be indirect or direct.

  Indirect injuries from stab or gunshot wounds and road accidents are rare. Commonest cause of ureteric injury is direct trauma (iatrogenic) during abdominal and pelvic operations.

  Both ureters are at risk during colonic and rectal surgery and gynaecological procedures. The left ureter is most commonly injured by the gynaecologist owing to its close proximity to the left vaginal fornix (p. 2).

Iatrogenic Trauma

1. Ligation of both ureters—anuria.
2. Ligation of one ureter—hydronephrosis and subsequent renal atrophy.
3. Leakage of urine from a divided ureter.
   Intraperitoneal:
   Abdominal distension, free fluid in peritoneal cavity and external leakage via drainage tube or abdominal incision.

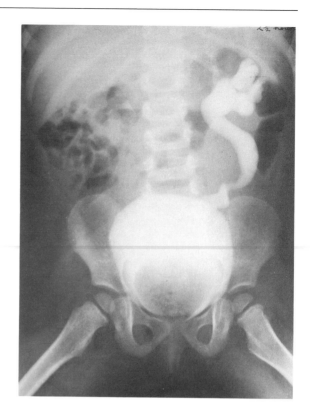

Extraperitoneal:
  Boggy mass in pelvis or loin and leakage via perineal wound or vagina in the female (vesico-vaginal fistula).

Clinical Features

1. Complete anuria—ligation of both ureters.
2. Intraperitoneal leakage of sterile urine—rapid pulse, pyrexia, abdominal tenderness and distension (ileus) with signs of free fluid in the abdominal cavity.
3. Intraperitoneal leakage of infected urine—peritonitis and septicaemia with rapid deterioration in patient's condition.
4. In 4, 5 or 6 days—fistula develops with drainage of urine from the wound or stab incision.
5. Extraperitoneal leakage—urine escapes from perineum or vagina.
6. Delayed leakage may occur 12–14 days after operation—due to damage to the ureteric blood supply.
7. Haematuria is invariably present after a ureteric injury.

Diagnosis

1. At time of operation—clear fluid collecting in the pelvic cavity.
2. Urgent IVU—non-function, hydroureter or leakage of dye from site of injury.

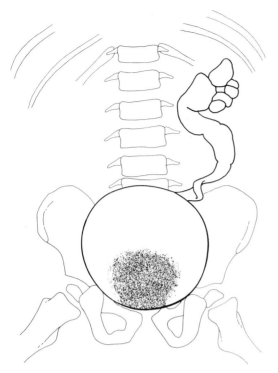

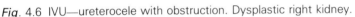

Fig. 4.6 IVU—ureterocele with obstruction. Dysplastic right kidney.

3.   Cystoscopy—blood efflux from damaged ureter.
4.   Retrograde ureterography—site of ligation or leakage from ureter identified.

Management
1.   At time of operation—immediate end-to-end repair over a splint or re-implantation into bladder (*Figs.* 4.7, 4.8).
2.   Within 7 days—immediate re-exploration: removal of mass ligatures and freeing of ureters. Transected ureter is repaired by end-to-end anastomosis (*Fig.* 4.7), or reimplantation into bladder (*Fig.* 4.8).
3.   Established fistula—3 weeks after operation—exploration and surgical repair as above.

Note:
   In critically ill patients—temporary percutaneous nephrostomy drainage. Following ureteric reconstruction for trauma a stricture may form three or four years after the original injury.

● **C. Inflammation of the Ureter**
   The ureteric urothelium becomes inflamed in acute pyelonephritis and cystitis, especially in the presence of reflux. Chronic inflammation of the ureter

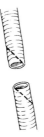
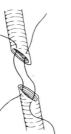
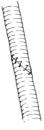

Incisions   'Trumpeting' of ends   Oblique anastomosis
of ureter

Fig. 4.7 End-to-end ureteric anastomosis.

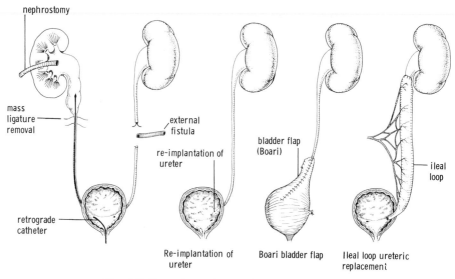

nephrostomy

mass
ligature
removal

external
fistula

re-implantation of
ureter

bladder flap
(Boari)

ileal
loop

retrograde
catheter

Re-implantation of   Boari bladder flap   Ileal loop ureteric
ureter   replacement

Fig. 4.8 Procedures for repair of ureteric injuries.

with fibrosis and stricture of its muscular wall may occur in chronic pyelonephritis and tuberculosis.

Retroperitoneal Fibrosis

In this chronic condition a dense sheet of fibrous retroperitoneal tissue extends laterally to encompass both ureters, often constricting the aorta and vena cava.

Aetiology
Unknown. Many patients will have a history of treatment for tuberculosis.

Clinical Features
Insidious in onset—uraemia, oliguria, abdominal and loin pains, backache and

ischaemic changes in the lower limbs due to constriction of the main abdominal vessels.

Diagnosis
1. Elevated ESR.
2. IVU:
    Deviation of middle third of both ureters towards midline with hydroureter and hydronephrosis above the compressed segment of ureter.

Treatment
1. Surgical:
    Liberation of constricted ureters from the surrounding fibrous envelope.
2. Anuria or oliguria:
    Urgent decompression of upper urinary tract by percutaneous nephrostomy and haemodialysis; subsequent definitive surgery for relief of ureteric obstruction.

●   **D. Ureteric Tumours**
    Malignant and benign tumours of the ureter are extremely rare.

Malignant Tumours
    Malignant tumours may be:
    Primary:
    Transitional cell urothelial carcinoma accounts for 1 per cent of all urothelial tumours.
    Secondary:
    Deposits from a primary tumour of the uterus, ovary, prostate and breast (adenocarcinoma).
    Direct involvement by extension from a carcinoma of the cervix, ovary, caecum, sigmoid colon and upper rectum.
    Note—the ureter is usually displaced or compressed by these tumours.

●   **E. Ureteric Dysfunction**
    Dysfunction of the ureteric musculature may produce the following clinical entities:
1. Obstructive muscular dysfunction:
        Upper ureter—congenital pelvi-ureteric obstruction.
        Lower ureter—simple megaureter.
2. Defective valvular mechanism:
        Lower ureter—vesico-ureteric reflux.

Congenital Pelvi-ureteric Obstruction

Aetiology and Pathology

A neuromuscular imbalance operates at the junction of the renal pelvis and ureter which will not allow peristaltic waves to pass distally. Internally the ureter has a mucosal flap, whilst externally the upper segment of ureter is kinked and tethered by fibrous peritoneal bands. An aberrant renal artery crosses the pelvi-ureteric junction in one third of patients. Secondary effects are hydronephrosis, pyonephrosis and stone formation (*Fig.* 4.9). The condition is bilateral in 20 per cent of patients.

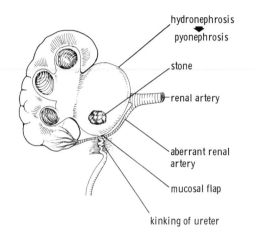

Fig. 4.9 Pathology of congenital pelvi-ureteric obstruction.

Clinical Features

In infancy, a visible and palpable renal mass is the commonest presenting feature.

In children and adults, recurrent urinary infection and haematuria are presenting symptoms. A palpable renal mass is found in 50 per cent of patients.

Investigations

1. Ultrasound scan:
   Differentiates between a solid and 'cystic' renal mass.
2. IVU demonstrates a large dilated renal pelvis with an abrupt 'shut-off' at the pelvi-ureteric junction (*Fig.* 4.10).
3. DTPA isotope scan:
   Assesses individual renal function and distinguishes between stasis and true obstruction at the pelvi-ureteric junction (*Fig.* 1.9).
4. Antegrade pyelography:
   This (p. 13) allows direct measurement of pressure within the renal pelvis and radiologically demonstrates obstruction to flow of dye from the pelvis into the upper ureter.

Treatment

1. Adults with mild obstruction, stasis and satisfactory renal function—no treatment.

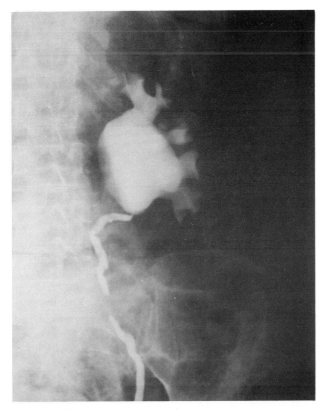

Fig. 4.10 Retrograde ureterography of pelvi-ureteric obstruction.

2. Infants, children and adults with obstruction and complications—operative treatment.
3. A non-functioning grossly hydronephrotic kidney—nephrectomy.
4. Operations of choice:
    Anderson–Hynes pyeloplasty (*Fig.* 4.11).
    Foley Y–V-plasty (*Fig.* 4.12).

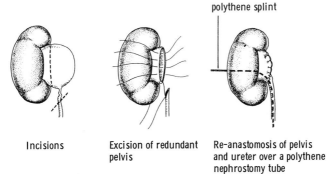

Incisions | Excision of redundant pelvis | Re-anastomosis of pelvis and ureter over a polythene nephrostomy tube

polythene splint

Fig. 4.11 Anderson–Hynes pyeloplasty.

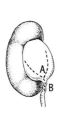 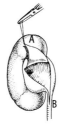

Incisions   Elevation of pelvic   Reconstitution of Y to V
                   flap

Fig. 4.12 Foley Y–V-plasty.

Simple (Primary) Megaureter

Aetiology and Pathology

1. A neuromuscular imbalance operates in the terminal ureter which acts as a block to the passage of peristaltic waves across the uretero-vesical junction.
2. The ureter proximal to the obstruction becomes dilated and hypertrophied.
3. The ureteric orifice is normal in shape and position with no vesico-ureteric reflux.
4. Two types of megaureter (*Fig.* 4.13) are recognized—short segment (90 per cent) and long segment (10 per cent).

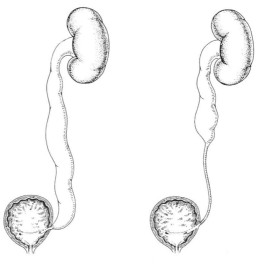

Short segment megaureter   Long segment megaureter

Fig. 4.13 Types of simple megaureter.

5. Condition is bilateral in 20 per cent.
6. Secondary hydronephrosis may develop: stones may form in the dilated ureter and renal pelvis.

Clinical Features
These include recurrent urinary tract infections and haematuria.

Investigations
1. Ultrasound:
   Dilatation of ureter.
2. IVU:
   Often normal renal pelvis with thickening and dilatation of ureter ending in a characteristic 'cone' at point of entry into bladder (*Fig.* 4.14). A thin-walled megaureter is tortuous.
3. Retrograde urography:
   Excessive peristalsis of the ureter observed on cine-radiography after retrograde injection of dye into the ureter.

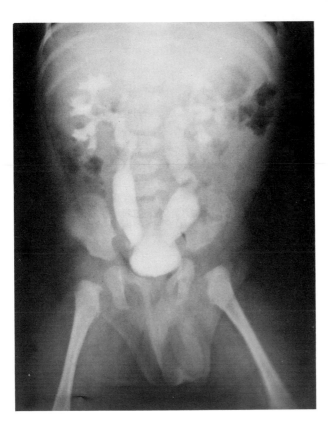

Fig. 4.14 IVU—simple megaureter.

Treatment

1. Mild degree of megaureter with normal renal function—no treatment.
2. Infection, stone formation or progressive hydronephrosis—operative treatment.
3. Thick-walled megaureter—trimmed and re-implanted into bladder—tunnel and cuff method (*Fig.* 4.20).
4. Thin-walled megaureter—trimmed and re-implanted using a reflux preventing procedure (*Fig.* 4.19).

Vesico-ureteric Reflux

Ureteric reflux may be primary (idiopathic) or secondary.

Secondary vesico-ureteric reflux results from increased pressure in the bladder due to bladder outlet or urethral obstruction and its management is surgery for relief of the obstruction.

Aetiology of Primary Reflux

1. Defective valvular mechanism at the uretero-vesical junction allows urine to reflux up to the ureter during increase in bladder pressure on micturition.
2. Congenital condition which manifests itself in childhood. Bilateral in 50 per cent.
3. 90 per cent of affected patients are female.

Pathology

1. The ureter either is normal in calibre or shows dilatation (refluxing megaureter).
2. The ureter enters the bladder in a horizontal direction, having lost its normal oblique intramuscular course (*Fig.* 4.15).

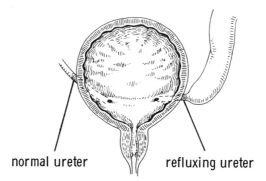

normal ureter   refluxing ureter

Fig. 4.15 Course of intramural ureter in reflux.

3. Affected ureteric orifice is patulous and wider than the normal orifice.
4. Infected urine will reflux to the kidney during micturition and may produce pyelonephritic changes and form stones.

Grading of Reflux

Four degrees of vesico-ureteric reflux are recognized depending on the extent of

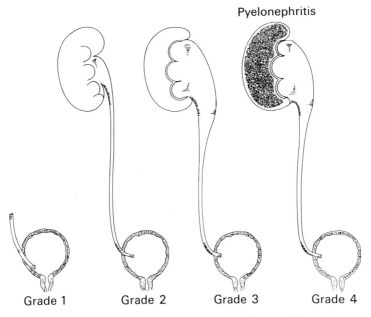

Pyelonephritis

Grade 1   Grade 2   Grade 3   Grade 4

Fig. 4.16 Radiological grading of ureteric reflux.

reflux demonstrated radiologically and the effect of reflux on the renal calices and parenchyma (*Fig.* 4.16).

Clinical Features
These include recurrent urinary tract infection and haematuria. Older children and adults may complain of pain in the loin on micturition.

Investigations
1.   IVU:
         Often normal or may show some hydroureter.
2.   Micturating cystogram:
         Demonstrates reflux and degree of reflux (*Fig.* 4.17).
3.   DTPA isotope scan:
         Demonstrates reflux and differential renal function (*Fig.* 4.18).
4.   DMSA static scan:
         Demonstrates parenchymal damage.

Treatment
Evidence exists to suggest that vesico-ureteric reflux is self-limiting and that children will grow out of their problems in their teens. Surgical treatment policy will depend on:
         Grade of reflux.
         Presence of recurrent infection.
         Evidence of renal scarring.
         Evidence of deterioration in renal function.

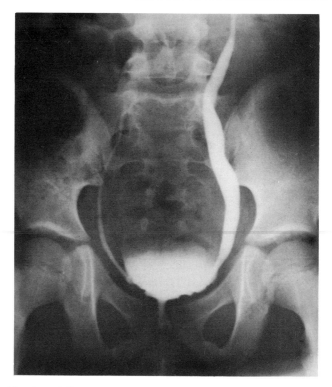

Fig. 4.17 Micturating cystography—idiopathic ureteric reflux.

1.   Grade I reflux—no treatment.
2.   Grade II reflux—no treatment: plus infection—long-term chemotherapy.
3.   Grade III reflux—plus or minus infection—surgical treatment.
4.   Grade IV reflux—surgical treatment.
      The operations of choice for ureteric re-implantation are the Politano-Leadbetter procedure (*Fig.* 4.19), and the Cohen operation.

Prognosis
Anti-reflux procedures are successful in preventing reflux in 90 per cent of patients. Bladder infections may persist after operation but should not have a deleterious effect on the kidney which is protected by the anti-reflux operation.

● **F. Hydronephrosis and Hydroureter**
      Hydronephrosis is a time-honoured term used to describe dilatation of the renal pelvis behind a distal obstruction. Hydroureter refers to a similar dilatation of one or both ureters. Pyonephrosis results from a secondary infection of an existing hydronephrosis.

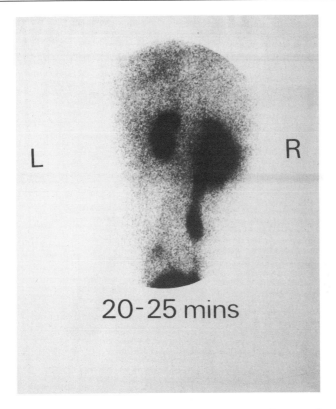

Fig. 4.18 DTPA isotope scan—dilated right ureter due to reflux.

Mechanics of Hydronephrosis and Hydroureter

The drainage system of the kidney may be regarded as a tubular structure with a dilated upper end (renal pelvis) leading to a narrow muscular tube (the ureter), which in turn opens into a capacious chamber (the bladder). The bladder voids its contents to the exterior via another muscular tube (the urethra). The ureter and urethra demonstrate points of natural narrowing along their course (*Fig.* 1.3) and pathological changes tend to occur at these points of narrowing. Being a tubular structure, the urinary drainage system may be constricted or obstructed in three ways:

1. Obstruction within the tube, e.g. stones.
2. Pathological changes in the wall of the tube, e.g. stricture, fibrosis, neoplasm.
3. Pressure from without the tube, e.g. extra-urogenital tumours.

The pathological processes which produce hydroureter and hydronephrosis will operate within one of these categories. A study of *Fig.* 4.21 will show that in unilateral hydronephrosis and hydroureter the obstructing lesion will occur between points A and B, whilst in bilateral hydronephrosis the obstruction will be between C and D.

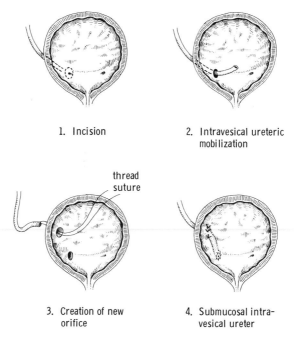

1. Incision

2. Intravesical ureteric
   mobilization

thread
suture

3. Creation of new
   orifice

4. Submucosal intra-
   vesical ureter

Fig. 4.19 Politano–Leadbetter ureteric re-implantation.

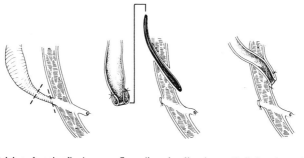

Division of ureter flush
with bladder wall

Formation of cuff and
oblique tunnel

Cuffed ureter sutured
inside bladder

Fig. 4.20 Tunnel-and-cuff method of ureteric re-implantation.

Aetiology

Unilateral Hydronephrosis and Hydroureter
1. Congenital:
    Pelvi-ureteric obstruction.
    Megaureter.
    Ureterocele.
2. Traumatic:
    Direct and indirect injury.
    Stricture following trauma or surgery.

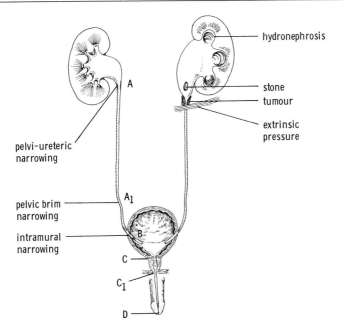

Fig. 4.21 Points of natural narrowing in urinary tract: common lesions producing obstructive uropathy.

3. Inflammatory:
    TB stricture.
    Stricture following stone impaction.
4. Stone.
5. Tumour:
    Primary or secondary ureteric tumour (rare).
    Tumour of bladder involving ureter.
6. Obstruction by extra-ureteric lesion, e.g. pelvic tumour or cyst.

Bilateral Hydronephrosis and Hydroureter
1. Congenital:
    Anterior and posterior urethral valves.
    Bladder neck stenosis.
    Ectopia vesicae.
2. Traumatic:
    Stricture after urethral rupture.
    Stricture after prostatectomy.
3. Inflammatory:
    Gonococcal stricture.
    TB stricture.
    Chronic prostatitis.
4. Tumours:
    Benign—prostatic hypertrophy (prostatomegaly).

Malignant:
  Bladder tumour.
  Carcinoma of the prostate.
  Extra-urogenital tumour:
    Uterine cervix.
    Rectum.
5. Neurogenic:
      Neuropathic bladder.
      Secondary vesico-ureteric reflux.

Pathology
1. Increasing pressure within the renal tract—distension of the renal pelvis (most obvious in an extra-renal pelvis).
2. Pressure in the renal calices—dilatation and stretching with change in contour from a 'cup shape' to 'club shape'.
3. Intra-pelvic and intra-caliceal pressure—pressure atrophy of adjacent parenchyma with loss of functioning nephrons.
4. Continued intra-pelvic pressure—renal enlargement—lobulated, cystic sac with a thin shell of parenchyma, representing the sole remains of functioning renal tissue (*Fig*. 4.22).

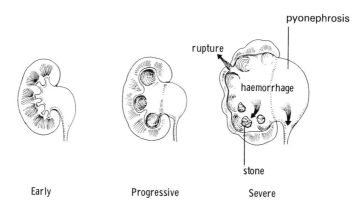

Fig. 4.22 Pathological changes in hydronephrosis.

Complications of Progressive Hydronephrosis
1. Secondary infection (pyonephrosis).
2. Stone formation.
3. Haemorrhage.
4. Rupture:
      Spontaneous.
      Trivial injury.
5. Hypertension—renal parenchymal ischaemia.
6. Renal failure.

Clinical Features

Unilateral Progressive Hydronephrosis
Often symptomless unless complications occur.
1. Pyonephrosis—toxic symptoms with a tender loin mass.
2. Stone formation—haematuria, dysuria and renal or ureteric colic.
3. Haemorrhage and rupture—loin pain and a palpable mass.
4. The hydronephrotic kidney will only be palpable in 50 per cent of patients.

Bilateral Progressive Hydronephrosis
Insidious in onset.
1. Anaemia in all patients.
2. Hypertension in a few patients.
3. Uraemia in all patients.
4. Chronic renal failure in long-standing chronic obstruction.

Investigations and Diagnosis of Obstructive Uropathy

Blood
Haemoglobin, ESR, urea estimation, bleeding and clotting times.

Urine
Examination for red cells, casts, pus cells and culture for organisms.

Radiology
1. Renal ultrasound scan:
   Often diagnostic and primary examination—echo-free area inside cortical kidney echoes.
2. Renal isotope scan:
   DTPA—differential renal function.
   DMSA—location and position of functioning renal parenchyma.
3. Antegrade pyelography:
   Site of obstruction.
   Pressure measurements within the renal pelvis.
4. IVU:
   Not helpful with grossly diminished renal function.
   'Delayed' films up to 24 hr indicated if secretion is not immediately evident on IVU.

Note:
   Functional excretion of contrast medium is possible until 60 per cent of nephrons in each kidney have been destroyed.

General Principles in Management of Obstructive Uropathy
   There are three main principles:
1. Relief of obstruction by external drainage or operation.
2. Elimination of infection in the urinary tract.
3. Conservation of functioning renal tissue.

Note:

Urinary tract obstruction and infection are a lethal combination in terms of rapid destruction of functioning nephrons and impairment of renal function.

Unilateral Obstruction

1. Obstruction *minus* infection *plus* good renal function—operative correction of obstruction.
2. Obstruction *plus* or *minus* infection *plus* poor renal function—nephrectomy.
3. Obstruction *plus* infection—urgent decompression by nephrostomy followed by:

    no function—nephrectomy.
    function—correction of obstruction.

Bilateral Obstruction

1. Obstruction *plus* or *minus* infection *plus* deteriorating renal function (uraemia):

    Urgent decompression by nephrostomy or bladder catheterization, *plus* or *minus* renal dialysis *plus* operative correction of obstruction when complete sterility and maximum recovery of renal function has been attained.
2. Oliguria or anuria:

    Renal dialysis *plus* early correction of obstruction.
    In advanced cases of chronic obstructive uropathy, where recovery of renal function cannot be achieved by decompression, renal dialysis will be continued and the patient considered for renal transplantation.

● **G. Operative Procedures on the Ureter**

The operations of nephrectomy and ureterolithotomy have been described in Chapters 2 and 3 (pp. 52 and 60). A partial nephrectomy combined with excision of the ureter in continuity (heminephroureterectomy) is employed in the treatment of ureteric duplication with pyelonephritic dysplasia of one half of the pyelon duplex (*Fig.* 4.3). The operations to be briefly described are pyeloplasty, ureteric anastomosis and ureteric re-implantation. Operative procedures for the repair of ureteric injuries are illustrated in *Fig.* 4.8 (p. 70).

Pyeloplasty

Two types of operation are commonly used:
1. For extra-renal pelvis—Anderson–Hynes pyeloplasty (*Fig.* 4.11).
2. For intra-renal pelvis—Foley Y–V-plasty (*Fig.* 4.12).

Anderson–Hynes Procedure

The upper ureter is transected obliquely, the stricture and redundant pelvis are excised and an anastomosis is fashioned over a nephrostomy splint.

Foley Procedure
A Y-shaped incision on front of the renal pelvis and upper ureter is converted to a V-shaped suture line.

Ureteric Anastomosis
Two ends of ureter are 'trumpeted' obliquely and anastomosed over a ureteric splint (*Fig.* 4.7).

Ureteric Re-implantation
Two basic operations are employed:
1. 'Tunnel and cuff' re-implantation for large ureters (*Fig.* 4.20).
2. Politano-Leadbetter re-implantation for normal or slightly dilated ureters (*Fig.* 4.19).

'Tunnel and Cuff' Procedure
The end of the ureter is trimmed to size and peeled back on itself to form a cuff. The cuffed ureter is re-implanted into the bladder.

Politano–Leadbetter Procedure
The ureter is dissected free from the bladder by a combined intra- and extra-vesical approach and re-implanted into the bladder in an oblique fashion within a muscular tunnel in the bladder wall.

Ureteric Replacement
In some patients a long segment of the ureter may be damaged or diseased. Complete replacement of the ureter is possible by the use of a viable loop of terminal ileum (*Fig.* 4.8).

5

The bladder

A. Congenital Anomalies of the Bladder

The bladder is formed from the urogenital sinus connected in early development to the umbilicus by a patent tube—the urachus. In the fully formed fetus the urachal duct is closed and disappears but may persist in the extra-peritoneal fat as a solid cord extending from the apex of the bladder to the umbilicus. Persistence of the duct produces a urachal fistula with leakage of urine at the umbilicus evident at birth. Failure of closure of the mid-portion of the urachus produces a urachal cyst palpable in the midline in the suprapubic region. Persistence of the bladder end of the urachus may be evident at cystoscopy as a urachal diverticulum at the fundus of the bladder (*Fig*. 5.1). The urinary bladder may rarely develop in two parts—double bladder—associated with urethral duplication. A congenital diverticulum may be found at cystoscopy, opening above and medial to the ureteric orifice and only rarely obstructing the juxtapositioned ureter.

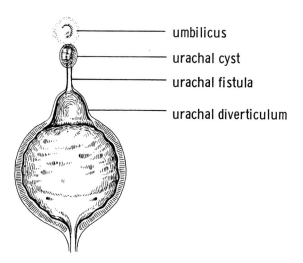

umbilicus

urachal cyst

urachal fistula

urachal diverticulum

Fig. 5.1 Urachal remnants.

Exstrophy of the Bladder (syn. Extroversion: Ectopia Vesicae)

Incidence
One in every 50 000 live births with equal sex incidence.

Pathology
Failure in development of the anterior wall of the urogenital sinus and of related skin and muscle of the lower abdomen. The posterior bladder wall, trigone and posterior urethra are laid open to the exterior and urine continually spills over the surrounding skin. Associated anomalies (*Fig.* 5.2) are

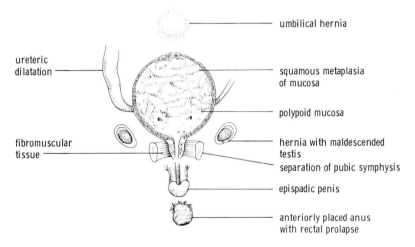

umbilical hernia

ureteric dilatation

squamous metaplasia of mucosa

polypoid mucosa

fibromuscular tissue

hernia with maldescended testis

separation of pubic symphysis

epispadic penis

anteriorly placed anus with rectal prolapse

Fig. 5.2 Exstrophy of bladder and associated anomalies.

1. Wide separation of the symphysis pubis.
2. Epispadias—the penis often being in two separate portions.
3. Umbilical and inguinal herniae.
4. Testicular maldescent.
5. Anterior placement of the anal orifice.
6. Rectal prolapse.
7. Occasionally extra-urogenital anomalies, e.g. atresia of oesophagus or duodenum. The exposed urothelium undergoes squamous metaplasia at the skin edges and may become polypoid in later years. The polypoid masses may undergo malignant change, producing an adenocarcinoma which is locally malignant and only rarely metastasizes. The untreated patient with exstrophy of the bladder rarely survives into adult life.

Management of Bladder Exstrophy
Parental distress dictates management policy in these patients. Definitive treatment is undertaken at the age of 6–9 months. IVU—assessment of upper urinary tract—rarely shows ureteric dilatation.
        Surgical treatment is reconstructive or diversionary.

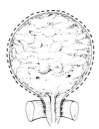 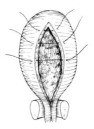 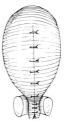

Incision – pubic bones   Mobilization of the bladder   Inversion and closure
approximated by osteotomy   of the bladder

Fig. 5.3 Bladder reconstruction in exstrophy of bladder.

Bladder Reconstruction (*Fig*. 5.3)
1. Bladder must be capacious with healthy mucosa.
2. Preliminary pelvic osteotomy to allow approximation of symphysis pubis.
3. In the male—penile reconstruction of epispadias at age of six or seven years.
4. Absence of sphincter muscles and nerve supply makes the reconstructed bladder an incontinent reservoir.
5. Operation removes the unsightly exstrophied bladder.

Results of Reconstruction
1. 60 per cent of girls—good, but may need intermittent self-catheterization.
2. 40 per cent of girls—poor, requiring urinary diversion.
3. 10 per cent of boys—good result.
4. 90 per cent of boys—poor and need diversion operation at an early age.

Urinary Diversion (Chapter 10, p. 175)
Excision of the bladder is combined with ureterosigmoidostomy (*Fig*. 10.6) or ileal or sigmoid loop conduit (*Fig*. 10.9).

Ureterosigmoidostomy is contraindicated in 40 per cent of infants with anal prolapse and defective anal musculature. It carries a 60 per cent risk of development of chronic renal failure due to ascending infection within 20 years of operation. Ileal or sigmoid loop conduit is operation of choice.

Recent Developments
Electronically controlled implant in bladder neck musculature may benefit some patients after bladder reconstruction.

● **B. Trauma to the Bladder**
Injuries to the bladder result from direct or indirect violence (*Fig*. 5.4):

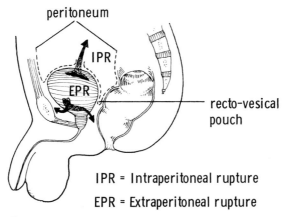

IPR = Intraperitoneal rupture

EPR = Extraperitoneal rupture

Fig. 5.4 Intra- and extra-peritoneal rupture of bladder.

1. Direct:
    Peroperative during abdominal or pelvic surgery—intraperitoneal.
    Endoscopic:
    Upper half of bladder—intra-peritoneal.
    Lower half of bladder—extra-peritoneal.
2. Indirect: external injury to lower abdomen
    Full bladder—intra-peritoneal leakage.
    Empty bladder—extra-peritoneal leakage.

Intra-peritoneal Rupture

Clinical Features
1. Sharp pain in lower abdomen at time of injury.
2. Increasing abdominal distension and discomfort (sterile urine).
3. Rapid development of signs of peritonitis (infected urine).
4. Attempts at micturition produce a few ml of blood-stained urine.
5. Anuria from time of injury.
6. Physical signs of ascites.

Diagnosis and Treatment
1. Catheterization under aseptic precautions in the operating theatre may produce a few ml of blood-stained urine.
2. Emergency operation:
    Laparotomy and cleaning of abdominal cavity.
    Repair of bladder laceration.
    Suprapubic catheterization.
    Antibiotic therapy.

Extra-peritoneal Rupture

Aetiology
1. Commonest cause is a fracture of the bony pelvis: associated with a urethral rupture in 40 per cent of cases.

2.   Iatrogenic injury:
            Per urethral resection.
            Pelvic and gynaecological surgery.
            Hernia operation, especially femoral hernia (bladder in posterior wall of hernial sac).

Presenting Symptoms
There is usually a history of:
1.   Trauma to bony pelvis.
2.   Gynaecological procedures—upper vaginal surgery.
3.   Pelvic surgery—rectal resections.
4.   Endoscopic resection of bladder—trigone and lateral walls.
            Extravasation of urine and blood into perivesical tissues produces a tender suprapubic mass and a tender boggy swelling on rectal examination.
            Repeated attempts at micturition produce small volumes of blood-stained urine.

Surgical Management
Clinical picture of oliguria, haematuria, suprapubic or pelvic mass and a history of external or operative trauma suggest a bladder injury. Immediate surgery is required:
1.   To decompress the bladder and drain extravasated fluid.
2.   Catheterization—preliminary to operation.
3.   Urethrography if integrity of urethra in doubt.
4.   Suprapubic exploration of the bladder and repair of injury if possible.
            Suprapubic bladder catheterization will provide drainage of extravasated fluid. Broad-spectrum antibiotic therapy may also be required.

• C. Infection of the Bladder: Bilharzia

Acute Cystitis
            Cystitis refers to hyperaemia and swelling of the bladder urothelium and is secondary to descending infection from the kidney or ascending infection from the urethra.

Aetiology
Cystitis is particularly prone to occur in females, in males with bladder outflow obstruction and in patients of both sexes with foreign bodies, calculi or tumours within the bladder. The common infecting organisms are *Escherichia coli*, *Bacillus proteus* and *Bacillus pyocyaneus*.

Clinical Features
Pyrexia and rigors, dysuria (pain on micturition), frequency, terminal haematuria and strangury—an intense but unsuccessful desire to micturate every few minutes. On examination the patient usually has suprapubic tenderness and tenderness within the pelvis on rectal and pelvic examination.

Diagnosis
1.   Clinical presentation.
2.   Ward examination of the urine—protein and blood.
3.   Laboratory examination of a clean sample of urine—red cells, epithelial débris and organisms.
4.   Urinary culture—isolation of infecting organism and sensitivity to a range of antibiotics.

Treatment
1.   Bed rest.
2.   Liberal fluid intake.
3.   Appropriate antibiotic, continued for 7 days after symptoms have subsided.

Chronic Cystitis

Aetiology
1.   Non-specific:
            Repeated attacks of acute cystitis.
            Inflammation in chronic pyelonephritis.
            Presence of foreign bodies, stones, fistulae and tumours in the bladder.
            Post-irradiation inflammation.
2.   Specific:
            Tuberculosis.
            Bilharziasis.

General Pathology
In long-standing specific and non-specific chronic cystitis the bladder urothelium may undergo squamous metaplasia (leukoplakia)—potentially a site for development of a squamous cell carcinoma. The bladder musculature becomes thickened by fibrosis which may result in a small-capacity contracted bladder.

Clinical Features
These include frequency, especially severe in a contracted bladder, with occasional dysuria and visible haematuria.

Diagnosis
1.   Ward examination of urine—always shows protein and blood.
2.   Laboratory examination of urine—epithelial débris, red cells, pus cells, but only rarely organisms.
3.   Cystoscopy and measurement of bladder capacity—often reduced to under 100 ml in a contracted bladder.
Note:
            In tuberculosis red cells and pus cells are present in urine but no infective organisms—sterile pyuria.

Treatment
1.   Specific medial treatment for tuberculosis and bilharziasis.

2. Long-term antibacterial therapy for non-specific chronic cystitis.
3. Operative treatment for foreign bodies, stones and tumours.
4. Enlargement of capacity of a contracted bladder by ileo- or colo-cysto-plasty (*Fig.* 5.23).

Bilharzia of the Bladder (syn. Schistosomiasis)
Genitourinary bilharziasis is caused by an infection by a blood fluke *Schistosoma haematobium*.

Aetiology
The main endemic areas are in the Middle East and East Africa particularly the Nile Valley and the Sudan. Modern air travel has led to an increase of reported cases in Western society.

Life Cycle
Definitive host—man. Paired adult worms produce ova in radicals of the pelvic and vesical veins. The ova migrate through the bladder wall into the urinary stream and hatch in fresh water to produce miracidia.

Intermediate host—the water snail. The miracidia penetrate the water snail and after 8 weeks small fork-tailed cercaria are released which penetrate the human skin and are carried in the blood stream to the pelvic venous plexuses where they develop into the adult fluke.

Pathology
Bladder lesions of bilharziasis are produced by inflammatory reaction to the presence of eggs in the bladder wall—secondary infection, fibrosis and calcification—small contracted bladder. Stone formation is common, and metaplastic changes in the urothelium may produce a squamous-cell carcinoma. The ureters and urethra may be involved in similar fibrotic lesions.

Symptoms
In the acute phase symptoms include pyrexia, urticaria, frequency, dysuria and haematuria. In the chronic phase—increasing frequency of micturition and haematuria.

Diagnosis
1. Identification of eggs in the urine and on rectal biopsy.
2. IVU—stone formation, strictures of the ureter, contraction of the bladder.
3. Cystoscopy—small bladder, bilharzial lesions around trigone, squamous metaplasia and frank malignancy.
4. Biopsy of bladder for histological confirmation.

Treatment
1. Medical—antimony tartrate.
2. Surgical:
   Removal of bladder stone.
   Excision of ureteric stricture.
   Enlargement of contracted bladder—ileo- or colo-cystoplasty (*Fig.* 5.23).

- ## D. Bladder Diverticulae: Bladder Fistulae

Bladder Diverticulum
    A diverticulum, is a flask-shaped urothelial protrusion through the muscle wall of the bladder. A diverticulum of the bladder may be congenital in origin, but most are acquired and associated with distal obstruction to the bladder outlet or urethra.

Aetiology
1.   Congenital diverticulum (*Fig.* 5.5):

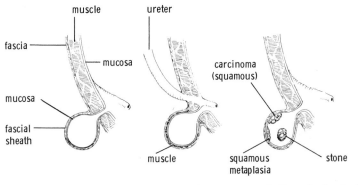

Acquired diverticulum   Congenital diverticulum   Complications of a diverticulum

Fig. 5.5 Bladder diverticula.

    Rare.
    Solitary and located medial to, and above, the ureteric orifice: urachal remnant diverticulum at apex of bladder (*Fig.* 5.1).
    Not associated with distal bladder outlet obstruction.
    Has muscle fibres within its wall and is contractile.
2.   Acquired diverticulum:
    Often multiple and located in the postero-lateral wall of the bladder.
    Always associated with distal obstruction, trabeculation and sacculation of the bladder.
    No muscle fibres in fundus, a flaccid fibrous sac, not emptying completely during micturition.
    Stagnation of urine in the diverticulum.
        Infection.
        Stone formation.
        Squamous metaplasia.
        Rarely, a squamous cell carcinoma.

Symptoms
There are no specific symptoms to indicate the presence of a diverticulum. Large diverticulae may fill with urine during the detrusor phase of micturition and

subsequently empty into the bladder to produce an immediate desire to pass urine a second time. Complicated diverticulae with infection, stones or tumour will give rise to frequency, dysuria and haematuria.

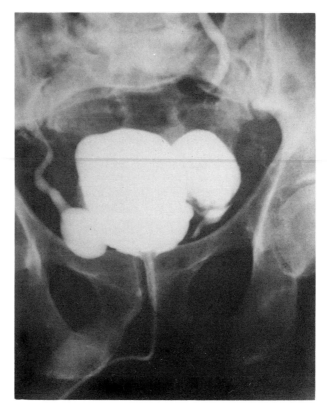

Fig. 5.6 Cystogram showing large diverticula in bladder outlet obstruction. Note reflux in both ureters.

Diagnosis

1. IVU—diverticulae readily seen during the cystogram phase of an IVU (*Fig.* 5.6).
2. Cystography and air-contrast cystography—visualization of interior of a diverticulum.
3. Cine-cystography—filling and emptying of a diverticulum visualized during micturition.
4. Cystoscopy—readily demonstrates diverticular openings within the bladder.

Treatment

1. Congenital diverticulum:
   Not excised unless producing ureteric obstruction.

2. Acquired diverticulum:
> Multiple small diverticulae with wide necks—no surgery.
> Solitary 'clean' diverticulum not producing ureteric obstruction—no surgery.
> 'Infected' diverticulum, containing stones, tumour or ureteric obstruction—operative treatment—diverticulectomy (*Fig.* 5.7).

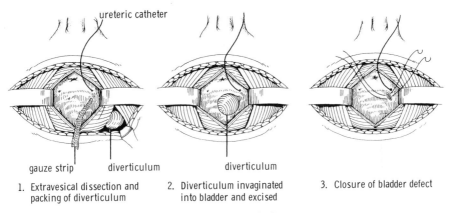

ureteric catheter

gauze strip diverticulum | diverticulum

1. Extravesical dissection and packing of diverticulum
2. Diverticulum invaginated into bladder and excised
3. Closure of bladder defect

Fig. 5.7 Bladder diverticulectomy.

Bladder Fistula
A fistula is a connecting epithelial-lined track, either between one hollow viscus and another or between a hollow viscus and the exterior.

Classification of Bladder Fistulae (*Fig.* 5.8)
1. Bladder to exterior:
> Congenital:
>> Urachal fistula (p. 86).
>> Exstrophy of bladder (p. 87).
> Acquired:
>> Suprapubic fistula.
>> Vesico-vaginal fistula.
2. Bladder to gut:
> Acquired:
>> Vesico-colic fistula.
>> Vesico-enteric fistula.
>> Vesico-rectal fistula.
3. Bladder to uterus:
> Acquired:
>> Vesico-uterine fistula.

Aetiology and Management
1. Suprapubic Fistula:
> Commonest cause is failure of closure of suprapubic incision after drainage of the bladder.

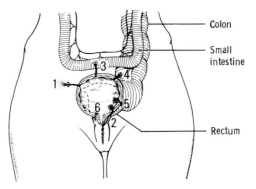

Fig. 5.8 Aetiology and pathology of bladder fistulae.
Key
1. Suprapubic—operative trauma: carcinoma.
2. Vesico-vaginal—operative trauma: carcinoma.
3. Vesico-enteric—Crohn's disease: carcinoma.
4. Vesico-colic—diverticulitis (75%): carcinoma (25%).
5. Vesico-rectal—trauma (prostatectomy): carcinoma.
6. Vesico-uterine—post-irradiation: carcinoma.

Fistula may persist after pelvic crush injuries.

Fistula may persist after operation on an infected or irradiated bladder.

Direct infiltration of a bladder tumour along the track of a suprapubic drain.

Treatment—excision and formal closure with perurethral catheter drainage for 12 days postoperatively.

2.   Vesico-vaginal Fistula:

Commonest cause is trauma to the bladder during difficult gynaecological procedures, e.g. total, Wertheim's or vaginal hysterectomy.

Direct extension of a carcinoma of the cervix into the bladder or a bladder carcinoma into the vaginal vault.

May follow irradiation treatment for carcinoma of the cervix or uterus.

Symptoms
Discharge of urine down the vagina and excoriation of the labia and thighs.

Diagnosis
1.   Methylene blue in bladder—leakage into vagina.
2.   Cystoscopy—visualization of bladder opening.
3.   IVU—to exclude damage to one or other ureter.

Treatment
1.   For non-malignant fistulae—surgical.
2.   Immediate repair is not advocated.
3.   After 6 weeks an established fistula is explored suprapubically, excised and closed in two layers (*Fig.* 5.9). Vesico-vaginal fistulae due to tumour

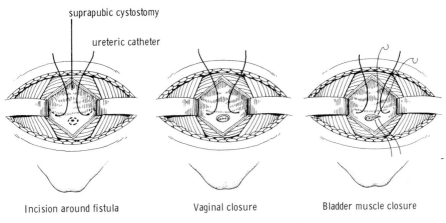

suprapubic cystostomy

ureteric catheter

Incision around fistula   Vaginal closure   Bladder muscle closure

Fig. 5.9 Repair of vesico-vaginal fistula.

infiltration or after irradiation are not suitable for excision and closure. For these patients a palliative urinary diversion by an ileal conduit or ureterosigmoidostomy is advised.

Fistula: Bladder to Gut

Direct attachment of bowel to bladder may result from inflammatory disease or a carcinoma of the bowel. Direct infiltration may establish a fistula, allowing gut contents and air to enter the bladder. Cystitis results and the patient will pass air bubbles (pneumaturia) and food debris in the urine during micturition.

1.   Vesico-enteric (small bowel) fistula:
            90 per cent—Crohn's disease.
            10 per cent—carcinoma.
2.   Vesico-colic (large bowel) fistula:
            75 per cent:
                    diverticulitis.
                    Crohn's disease.
                    ulcerative colitis.
            25 per cent—colonic carcinoma.
3.   Vesico-rectal fistula (rare):
            Iatrogenic—damage to rectal wall at prostatectomy.
            Rectal carcinoma infiltrating bladder.
            Bladder or prostatic carcinoma infiltrating rectum.

The commonest fistula is a vesico-colic connection due to diverticulitis, Crohn's disease or carcinoma of the sigmoid colon. This fistula typically involves the left side of the bladder fundus.

Diagnosis

1.   Diagnosis is seldom in doubt on clinical grounds—pneumaturia, débris and faeces in the urine.
2.   IVU, cystoscopy and barium enema—demonstrate the fistula (*Fig.* 5.10).

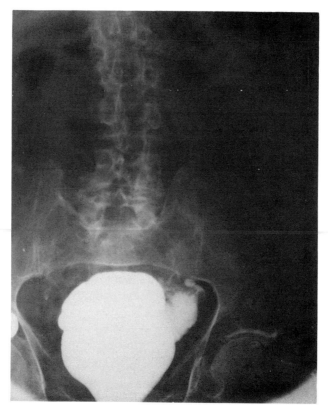

Fig. 5.10 Cystogram showing vesico-colic fistula—leakage of contrast medium into the pelvic colon.

3.   Cystoscopy and biopsy:
          Visualization of the bladder opening of the fistula.
          Biopsy—to exclude malignancy.

Treatment
1.   Surgical.
2.   Excision of fistula: closure of defect in bladder wall: resection of sigmoid colon, or small intestine.
3.   In a patient with a vesico-uterine fistula (rare) repair of the bladder is combined with a total hysterectomy.

●   **E. Neurogenic Dysfunction of the Bladder**
      Neurogenic dysfunction of the bladder results from either absence of, or interruption to, the reflex nerve pathways to the bladder and its sphincter muscles.

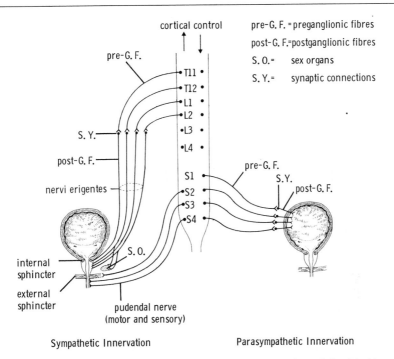

Fig. 5.11 Sympathetic and parasympathetic innervation of the bladder and its sphincter muscles.

Anatomy of Bladder Innervation

The act of normal micturition is governed by autonomic sympathetic and parasympathetic nerves. Parasympathetic nerves are concerned with function of the detrusor muscle, whilst sympathetic fibres influence function of the ureteric orifices, the bladder neck and sexual organs. The centres for parasympathetic control are in the second, third and fourth sacral segments of the spinal cord. Preganglionic fibres from these centres (S2, 3, 4) form the nervi erigentes and pelvic splanchnic plexuses which establish synaptic connections with peripheral ganglia outside or within the bladder detrusor muscle (*Fig.* 5.11). Sympathetic preganglionic fibres arise from the eleventh and twelfth thoracic and the first and second lumbar (T11, 12, L1, 2) segments of the spinal cord and establish synaptic connections within the spinal cord. Post-ganglionic sympathetic fibres reach the ureteric orifices, trigone and bladder neck along with the arterial blood supply. The external urethral sphincter is innervated by branches from the pudendal nerve (S2, 3, 4). Micturition is a reflex act involving the sympathetic and parasympathetic cord centres, but is influenced and partly controlled by higher centres in the cerebral cortex and mid-brain.

Physiology of Normal Micturition

Collection of urine within the bladder evokes a stretch reflex and impulses are transmitted via the parasympathetic nervi erigentes to the spinal centres (S1,

2, 3, 4) and at the same time to the cerebral cortex where the desire to micturate is consciously registered. The cerebral 'message' may be inhibited to a certain degree, but eventually cannot be suppressed and micturition becomes imperative. Autonomic impulses are released from the spinal centres which produce contraction of the detrusor muscle (parasympathetic) and concomitant relaxation of the internal sphincter (sympathetic). Voluntary contraction of the abdominal muscles and reflex relaxation of the pelvic floor muscles (pudendal nerve S2, 3, 4) facilitate expression of urine from the bladder. The presence of urine in the posterior urethra excites a further local reflex via the pudendal nerves, which maintains relaxation of the external sphincter to allow ejection of the last few drops of urine from the urethra.

Aetiology

The essential difference between neurogenic bladder dysfunction and bladder outlet obstruction is that in the latter the bladder and its sphincters are normally innervated.

Two categories of lesions are recognized in the aetiology of neurogenic bladder dysfunction:
1.   Traumatic:
        Spinal cord injuries.
        Operative trauma.
2.   Non-traumatic:
        Congenital:
            Myelomeningocele.
            Sacral agenesis.
            Spina bifida occulta.
        Acquired:
            Extradural abscess.
            Spinal tuberculosis.
            Cerebrovascular accidents.
            Tabes dorsalis (syphilis).
            Subacute combined degeneration of cord.
            Disseminated sclerosis.
            Prolapsed intervertebral disc.
            Spinal tumours.
            Sacral tumours.

Clinical Features

Patients with a neurogenic bladder fall into three aetiological groups—congenital, traumatic and acquired.

Congenital Neurogenic Bladder

A congenital neurogenic bladder is always associated with a spinal defect due to failure in development of the posterior vertebral arches with or without a defect of the neural tube. Three varieties of spinal and cord defect are recognized with descending order of severity:
1.   Myelomeningocele (95 per cent of spina bifida cases)—exposed cystic swelling in the midline over the lumbar spine and sacrum or rarely over the thoracic spine. The sac contains cerebrospinal fluid and the neural plate,

nerve roots and spinal cord. Innervation of the lower limbs is defective (paraplegia) and in 80 per cent there is a developing hydrocephalus due to increase in pressure of cerebrospinal fluid in the spinal canal. In 20 per cent of patients other anomalies are evident in the genito-urinary tract —multicystic or horseshoe kidneys, hypospadias and testicular maldescent.

2. Meningocele (5 per cent of spina bifida cases)—flat swelling over the spinal cord with normal skin covering, containing cerebrospinal fluid and no nerve elements.

3. Spina bifida occulta—defective fusion of vertebral arches of fifth lumbar and first sacral vertebrae. The overlying skin may show a dermal pit, a hairy patch or a fibro-fatty lump with skin discoloration.

Incidence
Spina bifida occulta and meningomyelocele occur in 3·5 per 1000 live births in the United Kingdom.

Diagnosis
The congenital anomaly in the spinal cord is evident at birth in most instances. A spina bifida occulta may cause problems if the overlying skin is normal in appearance and there is no evident swelling over the spinal cord. Absence of perineal sensation is a useful diagnostic sign in some of these patients. The bladder dysfunction is of three types:

1. Inert bladder:
No sensation, no detrusor activity, no outflow resistance—incontinence.

2. Uncoordinated reflex bladder:
Strong detrusor activity, failure of relaxation of internal sphincter, high pressure bladder with overflow incontinence—reflux— hydronephrosis—chronic renal failure.

3. Coordinated reflex bladder:
Bladder function controlled by spinal bladder centre (S2, 3, 4) —'automatic' and complete emptying is achieved—a rare phenomenon.

IVU will demonstrate obstructive uropathy in the uncoordinated reflex bladder.

Urodynamic studies (p. 18) in older age group will demonstrate uncoordinated detrusor activity with high intra-vesical pressure.

Management
Objectives in the management of a neurogenic bladder are:

1. Prevention of infection in the urinary tract.
2. Preservation of upper tract function.
3. Control of urinary incontinence.

The inert and the coordinated reflex bladder patients require no treatment in infancy. In later years intermittent self-catheterization by the parent or child or a permanent indwelling catheter in girls and a penile urine collecting bag in boys may manage the incontinence. Signs of upper urinary tract infection and deterioration of renal function are indications for urinary diversion. The uncoordinated reflex bladder may be managed by intermittent hourly catheterization, but infection and upper tract deterioration usually rapidly supervene and urinary diversion at an early stage is advocated.

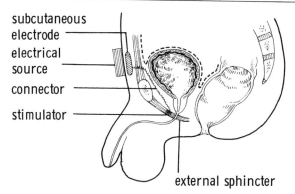

subcutaneous
electrode
electrical
source
connector
stimulator

external sphincter

Fig. 5.12 Method of electrical stimulation of external bladder sphincters.

Traumatic Neurogenic Bladder

Transection of the spinal cord above the bladder spinal autonomic centres will produce paraplegia and bladder dysfunction. In the state of spinal shock, lasting 1 week to 3 months, the bladder becomes overdistended (painless) and empties by overflow. Return of function to the bladder spinal reflex centres (S2, 3, 4) will produce an automatic or cord bladder which empties involuntarily every two or three hours. An established cord bladder is frequently compromised by infection, stone formation, ureteric reflux, hydronephrosis, chronic pyelonephritis and amyloidosis.

Management

The patients are treated in a spinal injury centre.
1. Early treatment—in both sexes—intermittent self-catheterization.
2. Later treatment:
    In male patients:
    Incontinent—condom type of urinal.
    Retention:
    Perurethral sphincterotomy converting retention to incontinence.
    In female patients:
    Incontinent—urinary diversion.
    Retention:
    Suprapubic expression of bladder.
    Permanent catheterization.
    In both sexes—failure of above methods of management, persistent urinary tract infection, deterioration of renal function are indications for urinary diversion.

Acquired Neurogenic Bladder

1. Insidious in presentation.
2. Multiple aetiology.
3. Cord or automatic bladder never develops in these patients.
4. Presenting urological complaint:
    Retention with overflow.
    Incontinence of urine.

5. Managed on the same lines as described above for the established paraplegic bladder.

Future Developments
Stimulators implanted in the bladder sphincter muscles are activated by a power source fixed externally over the lower abdomen (*Fig.* 5.12). Constant stimulation by the electrodes may restore a degree of sphincter control to the muscles of the bladder outlet and prostatic urethra.

● **F. Incontinence of Urine: The Unstable Bladder**

Incontinence

Definition
Incontinence is involuntary passage of urine from the urethra.

Normal Continence of Urine
Urinary continence is maintained by two muscle groups, the internal sphincter, surrounding the bladder neck, which is involuntary, and the external sphincter, surrounding the distal prostatic urethra, which is voluntary (*Fig.* 5.13). In the male a third group of involuntary muscle fibres—intrinsic urethral sphincter—are incorporated in the wall of distal third of the prostatic urethra and produce retrograde emptying of urine from the prostatic urethra on completion of micturition. The internal sphincter in normal circumstances is capable of maintaining continence of urine. If the internal sphincter is disrupted or defective, the external sphincter can maintain continence.

Development of Urinary Continence
A normal infant will be dry in day-time by the age of 18 months, whilst napkins at night cannot be discarded with confidence until the child is two or three years of age. Late development of reflex control of micturition from higher centres may delay the attainment of complete continence at night for a further 12–18 months.

Aetiology
Incontinence may be functional or organic in origin.
1. Functional:
    Enuresis.
    Giggle incontinence.
2. Organic:
    Congenital:
        Ectopic ureter (p. 63).
        Exstrophy of bladder (p. 87).
        Epispadias.
        Sacral teratomas.

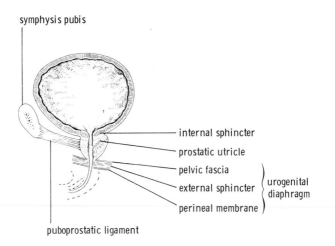

symphysis pubis

internal sphincter
prostatic utricle
pelvic fascia
external sphincter ⎱ urogenital
⎰ diaphragm
perineal membrane

puboprostatic ligament

Fig. 5.13 Sphincter muscles of the bladder outlet and urethra.

Traumatic:
    Childbirth.
    Pelvic crush injuries.
    Prostatectomy and bladder neck surgery.
    Gynaecological and vaginal surgery.
Mechanical:
    Benign and malignant disease of prostate gland.
    Uterine prolapse.
Neurogenic:
    Myelomeningocele.
    Spinal cord injuries.
    Spinal cord tumours.
    Neurological disease.

Functional Incontinence
Enuresis refers to childhood incontinence occurring without demonstrable evidence of neurological or urological pathology. Sufferers wet the bed at night (nocturnal enuresis) but may also wet in the daytime (diurnal enuresis). There is often a strong family history of bed-wetting. The condition is self-limiting, few patients being affected after puberty.

Aetiology is unknown. Cortical stimulation to micturate is inhibited, whilst the bladder itself is hypersensitive to distension which leads to precipitate micturition. Psychological factors may operate—nail biting has been observed in 17 per cent of patients. There are no organic changes in the bladder and urethra to account for enuresis and clinical examination and investigation are normal. The act of micturition is normal.

Treatment is along medical lines using reassurance and counselling, bladder training, drug therapy (imipramine), and night alarm bells in recalcitrant cases. In a few patients, hospital admission and a cystoscopy may cure the complaint.

Giggle incontinence is a rare condition affecting girls, who have normal bladder control, but are unable to prevent themselves completely emptying the bladder on giggling or laughing. The condition is familial and there is no effective treatment.

Organic Incontinence

The aetiological factors in organic incontinence are enumerated above. True incontinence from congenital causes is described on p. 64, and neurogenic incontinence and its management on p. 100. The incontinence produced by a congenital or neurogenic lesion is complete in that there is no bladder sensation and no control over the loss of urine from the bladder. Incontinence from a mechanical or traumatic cause is partial in nature, the patient being aware that urine is leaking down the urethra. The various forms of partial incontinence of urine of mechanical origin are as follows:

1. Terminal incontinence—occurs in middle-aged and elderly males and is due to retention of a small amount of urine in the bulbar urethra below the external sphincter. This urine leaks to the exterior after micturition. The retained urine may be manually expressed by perineal massage, thus avoiding wetting of underclothes after micturition.

2. Urge incontinence—inability of the patient with prostatomegaly to get to the toilet in time to empty the bladder.

3. Stress incontinence—leakage of urine from the female urethra during increase in abdominal pressure on straining, laughing or sneezing: common in females after childbirth and the result of weakness of the pelvic floor muscles (cystocele and rectocele). Treated by a repair operation and in unsuccessful cases by a urethral buttress or sling procedure.

4. Overflow incontinence—occurs in patients in chronic urinary retention with a large distended bladder (p. 125).

5. Small bladder syndrome—patients with a small capacity bladder (tuberculous cystitis: bilharzia) have severe frequency and incontinence of urine due to inability of the bladder to distend and hold urine. Treatment is operative to enlarge the bladder capacity by an ileo- or colo-cystoplasty (p. 117).

Diagnosis and Investigation of Incontinent Patients

Incontinence will be clinically evident from the patient's complaints combined with a uriniferous odour, soiled underclothes and excoriation of the skin over the external genitalia and inner thighs. IVU demonstrates the upper tract and evidence of post-micturition residual urine in patients with bladder outflow obstruction. Urodynamic studies and urethral pressure profiles are useful adjuncts in investigating incontinent patients, as they demonstrate both detrusor and urethral sphincter activity (*Fig.* 1.12).

Management of Incontinence

The management of incontinence from various aetiological causes is discussed in relevant sections of the book and are listed on the classification chart of incontinence (p. 103). Incontinence due to bladder outflow obstruction is often cured by surgical treatment of the obstructive lesion, e.g. prostatectomy. A group of male and female patients in the traumatic and mechanical groups remain incontinent, and in these patients electrical control of the bladder sphincters may be appropriate. Electrical impulses are transmitted to the implanted stimulator in the sphincter muscles from a subcutaneous electrode sited in the lower abdominal region and triggered from the exterior by a battery worn around the patient's waist (*Fig.* 5.12).

The Unstable Bladder (syn. Bladder Instability)

Bladder instability is a condition in which uncoordinated detrusor contractions occur in an otherwise normal lower urinary tract.

Aetiology

Aetiology is unknown.

Clinical Features

The condition occurs in middle-aged females with a psychogenic background. Symptoms include frequency, nocturia, dysuria and urge incontinence.

Diagnosis

1. Clinical examination of the patient reveals no abnormality.
2. At cystoscopy the bladder is normal.
3. IVU is normal.
4. Urodynamic studies—filling cystometry and voiding pressure flow studies—positive diagnosis.
5. Filling cystometry—phasic increases in pressure during filling as compared with a gradual rise of pressure in the normal bladder (*Fig.* 1.12).
6. Voiding studies—similar uncoordinated detrusor contractions are seen during the voiding phase of micturition.

Treatment

There is no universal treatment for bladder instability. Antihistamine drugs, urethral dilatation, bladder distension (Helmstein), bladder denervation and operations for enlarging bladder capacity (ileo- or colo-cystoplasty) have all been tried with varying degree of success in the management of this condition.

● G. Bladder Tumours

Bladder tumours may arise from the muscular wall and connective tissue or from the urothelium (transitional cell carcinoma). Primary tumours of the bladder muscle, benign and malignant, are extremely rare—fibroma, leiomyoma, leiomyosarcoma, rhabdomyosarcoma (malignant tumour of childhood). The bladder muscle may rarely be the site of secondary metastases of a distant primary tumour of the ovary, bowel, pancreas or bronchus. The bladder is not infrequently involved by direct secondary spread from a malignant tumour of adjacent pelvic organs—rectum, colon, small intestine, ovary, uterus and cervix—the tumours are adenocarcinomata or squamous cell carcinomata.

Tumours of the Bladder Urothelium
1.   Benign tumours:
             Papilloma—1 per cent.
2.   Malignant tumours:
             Transitional cell—95 per cent.
             Squamous cell and
             Adenocarcinoma—4 per cent.

Incidence of Urothelial Tumours
Bladder cancer accounts for 5 per cent of cancer mortality in Britain, whilst in Egypt and the Middle East, where bilharzia is a common bladder infection, the figure is 15 per cent. The incidence of bladder carcinoma has shown a steady increase in Britain over the past decade. Bladder carcinoma presents in the sixth and seventh decades with a $5:1$ male preponderance.

Aetiology of Bladder Carcinoma
1.   Carcinogens excreted in urine—aniline, 2-naphthylamine, benzidine and xenylamine.
2.   Workers at risk—dye, chemical, printing and rubber industries.
3.   Risk factor—40 times greater risk for these workers compared with other industrial occupations.
4.   Ectopic bladder—adenocarcinoma after many years of exposure.
5.   Bilharzial bladder—malignant changes—44 per cent are squamous cell carcinoma.
6.   Bladder stasis—may predispose to malignant change in urothelium.
7.   Smoking—may predispose to malignancy.
Note:
      Continued excretion of carcinogens in the urine after adequate treatment of a urothelial carcinoma accounts for the frequency of recurrence of tumours.

Pathology and Staging of Urothelial Tumours (*Fig.* 5.14)
All urothelial tumours must be regarded as potentially malignant:
1.   Transitional cell carcinoma   —95 per cent.
2.   Squamous cell carcinoma   — 3 per cent.
3.   Primary adenocarcinoma   — 1 per cent.
4.   Benign papilloma   — 1 per cent.
      The tumour may present as:
1.   A flat plaque in the urothelium—carcinoma in situ.
2.   Pedunculated lesion—papilloma and papillary tumour.
3.   Sessile tumour.
4.   Ulcerating tumour—malignant ulcer.

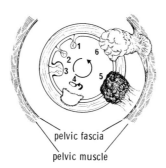

1. 'Papilloma'
2. Papillary carcinoma
3. Solid carcinoma
4. Malignant ulcer
5. Infiltrating tethered tumour
6. Infiltrating fixed tumour

pelvic fascia

pelvic muscle

Fig. 5.14 Pathological types of bladder carcinoma.

5.   Solid mass—solid carcinoma.

About 70 per cent of tumours arise in the posterior and postero-lateral walls of the bladder.

Histological Grading

Histologically, the tumour cells show varying degrees of differentiation correlated with invasiveness of the tumour, its local spread and its tendency to metastasize to regional lymph nodes and to other organs in the body.

Grading:

1.   G0—papilloma: no malignant change.
2.   G1—well differentiated.
3.   G2—moderate differentiation.
4.   G3—undifferentiated (anaplastic).

A single tumour may contain a mixture of well-differentiated and anaplastic cells.

Tumour Staging

The earliest detectable malignant change in the urothelium is a carcinoma in situ—a flat reddish plaque on the urothelium. A bladder tumour is staged by the degree of invasion into the bladder musculature and direct spread and fixation to surrounding structures.

1.   TIS—carcinoma in situ.
2.   T1—papilloma and papillary carcinoma—has not invaded beyond the lamina propria.
3.   T2—solid, sessile or ulcerating lesion—invasion beyond the lamina propria.
4.   T3—ulcerating tumour through bladder wall—not tethered.
5.   T4—solid or ulcerating tumour with tethering and fixation to surrounding structures and pelvic wall.

A carcinoma of the bladder metastasizes to the lymph nodes and by the blood stream:

Lymphatic spread:

To the lymph nodes adjacent to the bladder wall.

To internal iliac nodes.

To para-aortic nodes.

To lymph nodes at distant sites.

Lymph node staging is made peroperatively as the involved nodes are not accessible to clinical palpation.

Lymph node staging (peroperative: histological):

N0—no nodes involved.

N1—single regional node.

N2—multiple regional nodes.

N3—fixed regional nodes.

N4—distant lymph nodes involved.

Blood-stream spread:

Liver.

Lungs.

Long bones.

Other organs.

Staging:

M0—no metastases.

M1—distant blood-borne metastases.

Clinical Features

1. Painless haematuria—80 per cent.
2. Dysuria with or without haematuria—12 per cent.
3. Prostatism or 'silent' presentation—8 per cent.

Clinical examination is unrewarding in most patients. Distant metastases in the liver, lungs or bones is the method of presentation in 5 per cent of patients. Suspect a carcinoma of the bladder in a male between the ages of 50 and 80 who presents with painless haematuria. Advanced cases present with suprapubic and perineal pain with severe dysuria, strangury and continual leakage of offensive blood-stained urine from the urethra.

Diagnosis

Urothelial tumours are often multicentric in origin and complete assessment of the urinary tract from the calices to the urethra is essential in all patients.

1. Urine culture and microscopy:

    Evidence of secondary infection.

    Microscopic haematuria.

2. Urine cytology:

    Malignant cells.

3. Blood examination:

    Anaemia and elevated ESR.

4. Blood urea and creatinine:

    Uraemia and renal failure in advanced disease.

5. IVU:

    Filling defect in cystogram phase (*Fig.* 5.15), ureteric obstruction, evidence of other urothelial tumours in the urinary tract.

6. Cystourethroscopy:

    Type, size, position and number of bladder tumours.

    Biopsy and histological grading in all tumours.

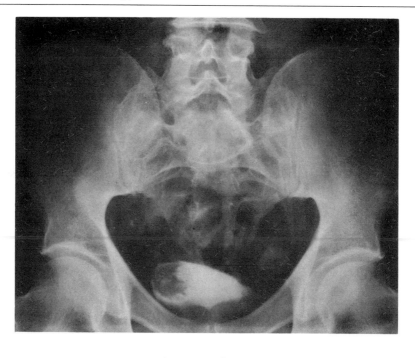

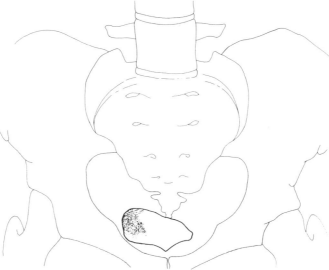

Fig. 5.15 Cystogram: filling defect due to a bladder carcinoma.

7.   Bimanual examination:
        Under complete relaxation and a general anaesthesia—tumour
        palpated and tethering or fixation to surrounding structures assessed.
8.   Ultrasonography:
        Full bladder (echo free): tumour is echogenic and an accurate
        assessment of infiltration of the bladder wall is possible in 80 per cent.

9. Chest X-ray and bone scan:
   Detection of distant metastases.
10. Lymphography:
    Detection of involvement of iliac and para-aortic lymph nodes.
11. CT scan:
    If available—detection of secondary intra-abdominal lymph node metastases.

The four essential examinations in assessment of a bladder tumour are an IVU, cystourethroscopy, bimanual examination of the bladder and tumour and biopsy for histological grading. With the information available from these investigations TNM staging of the tumour is undertaken and the success of treatment and the patient's prognosis will ultimately depend on the accuracy of staging (*Fig.* 5.16).

Treatment

The treatment policy for urothelial bladder carcinoma is dependent upon the site, number, size and histological grading of the tumour. Anaplastic (G3) tumours are treated by radiotherapy initially, whatever their size or number. G1 and G2 tumours are treated by a combination of surgery and radiotherapy. The methods available for treating bladder carcinoma fall into three categories:

1. Endoscopy:
   Endoscopic operations.
   Cystodiathermy.
   Perurethral resection.
2. Surgery:
   Ablative operations:
   Partial cystectomy.
   Total cysto-prostatectomy.
   Palliative operations:
   Ureterosigmoidostomy.
   Urinary conduit.

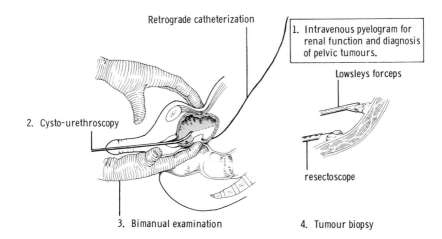

Retrograde catheterization

1. Intravenous pyelogram for renal function and diagnosis of pelvic tumours.

Lowsleys forceps

2. Cysto-urethroscopy

resectoscope

3. Bimanual examination

4. Tumour biopsy

Fig. 5.16 Four diagnostic methods for assessing a bladder tumour.

3.   Radiotherapy and chemotherapy:
         External radiotherapy.
         Intracavitary chemotherapy.
         Tumour infusion with cytotoxic agents.
4.   Combined surgery and radiotherapy:
         Endoscopic gold seed implantation.
         Transvesical gold seed implantation.

         Selection of treatment is dependent on tumour staging:
1.   Carcinoma in situ (TIS):
         Endoscopic diathermy or resection: intracavitary chemotherapy: if
         invasive (G3) radical surgery.
2.   T1:
         Single—cystodiathermy or endoscopic resection.
         Multiple—intracavitary chemotherapy.
         Recurrent—cysto-prostatectomy.
3.   T2:
         Single—endoscopic resection or gold seed implant.
         Multiple—external radiotherapy.
         Recurrent—partial cystectomy (single) cystoprostatectomy
         (multiple).
4.   T3:
         Primary treatment—radiotherapy.
         Recurrent tumour—cystoprostatectomy.
5.   T4:
         Palliative radiotherapy.
         Palliative urinary diversion.
Note:
         Cystoprostatectomy, either radical or palliative, is often indicated for
         bleeding and contraction of the bladder following primary treatment of a
         tumour by radiotherapy. The primary treatment for a bladder carcinoma in
         the majority of patients is endoscopic resection. Bladder tumours have a
         multicentric origin and are prone to recurrence in the bladder. T1 and T2
         tumours have a 50 per cent incidence of recurrence or new tumour
         formation (multicentric). Regular follow-up by cystoscopy two or three
         times a year is essential in bladder tumour patients, often for a period of up
         to 10 years following primary treatment.

Urine Cytology
1.   Microscopic examination of urine for malignant cells.
2.   Screening for treated bladder cancer patients: valueless in the irradiated
      bladder.
3.   Routine annual screening of industrial workers at risk—dye, chemical,
      printing and rubber industries.

Prognosis
   Invasive carcinoma in situ (TIS) has a good prognosis. Poorly differentiated and anaplastic tumours (G3) have a poor prognosis:

T1—75 per cent 5-year survival.
T2—37 per cent 5-year survival.
T3—radiotherapy + radical surgery—20 per cent 5-year survival.
T4—average survival after radiotherapy + or − palliative surgery is 6 months.

- **H. Operations on the Bladder**
  There are two types of operation:
  > Endoscopic procedures.
  > Open (per abdominal) operations.

Endoscopic Procedures
1. Retrograde catheterization.
2. Cystodiathermy (*Fig.* 5.17).
3. Perurethral resection (*Fig.* 5.18).
4. Internal urethrotomy and bladder neck incision (*Fig.* 6.5).

Open Operations
  The commonest surgical procedure on the bladder is a suprapubic

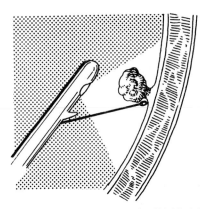

Fig. 5.17 Diathermy coagulation of a T1 bladder tumour.

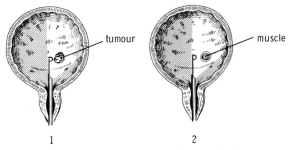

Fig. 5.18 Endoscopic resection of a T2 bladder tumour.

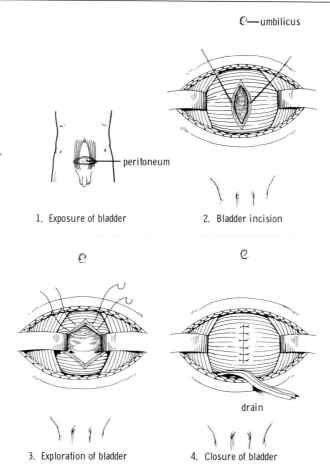

Fig. 5.19 Suprapubic cystotomy.

cystotomy (*Fig.* 5.19). The bladder is approached by a midline or transverse suprapubic incision opening into the retropubic space extraperitoneally. The cystotomy incision is made on the anterior wall of the vault of the bladder.

Operative Procedures via Cystotomy
1. Partial cystectomy (*Fig.* 5.21).
2. Open bladder neck resection.
3. Diverticulectomy (*Fig.* 5.7).
4. Y–V-plasty of bladder neck (*Fig.* 6.6).
5. Vesico-colic or vesico-vaginal fistula repair (*Fig.* 5.9).
6. Open resection of bladder tumour and gold seed implant (*Fig.* 5.20).
Note:

After closure of the cystotomy incision bladder drainage is maintained by a urethral catheter for 7–10 days and the retropubic space is drained for 3–5 days.

tumour excised to muscle

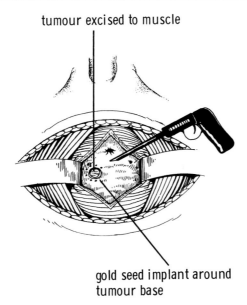

gold seed implant around
tumour base

Fig. 5.20 Open radioactive gold seed implant into a T2 bladder tumour (total dosage 6000 rads).

Operations for Bladder Tumours
1. Cystodiathermy (*Fig.* 5.17).
2. Endoscopic resection:
    Treatment of choice for majority of T1 and T2 tumours (*Fig.* 5.18).
3. Radioactive gold seed implant:
    Open operation (*Fig.* 5.20).
    Endoscopic.
4. Partial cystectomy (*Fig.* 5.21):
    Suitable only for solitary T2 tumours in vault of bladder.
5. Total cystectomy (*Fig.* 5.22):

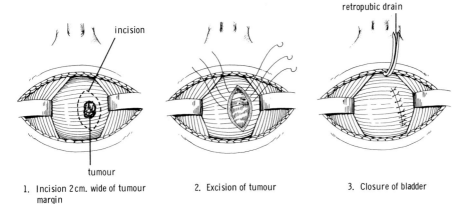

incision

retropubic drain

tumour

1. Incision 2 cm. wide of tumour margin

2. Excision of tumour

3. Closure of bladder

Fig. 5.21 Partial cystectomy.

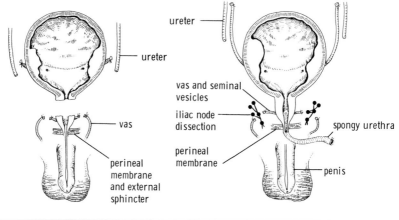

ureter

ureter

vas and seminal vesicles

iliac node dissection

perineal membrane

spongy urethra

penis

vas

perineal membrane and external sphincter

TOTAL CYSTECTOMY

RADICAL CYSTECTOMY

Fig. 5.22 Total cystectomy: radical cystoprostatectomy.

Palliative removal of T2 or T3 tumours with metastases or for post-irradiation contracted bladder.

6. Radical cysto-prostatectomy (*Fig*. 5.22):
Primary treatment for a T2 or T3 tumour confined to the bladder, combined with pre- or postoperative radiotherapy.

Note:
Total and radical cystectomy will involve a urinary diversion, usually an ileal loop conduit.

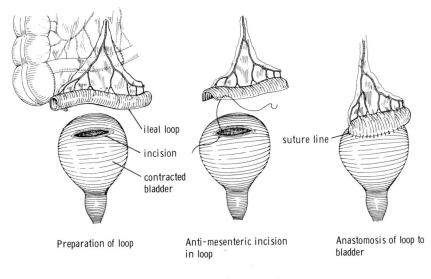

ileal loop

incision

contracted bladder

suture line

Preparation of loop

Anti-mesenteric incision in loop

Anastomosis of loop to bladder

Fig. 5.23 Ileocystoplasty.

Operations for enlargement of bladder capacity are used for the small contracted bladder found in tuberculosis, chronic cystitis and bilharzia. A vascularized loop of ileum, colon or caecum is anastomosed to the fundus of the bladder (*Fig*. 5.23).

6

The prostate gland

- **A. Prostatic Anatomy and Physiology**

The prostate gland occupies a unique position in the male genito-urinary tract, lying at the point of confluence of the genital and urinary conduits and closely related posteriorly to the rectum. Pathological conditions of the prostate gland may therefore produce functional disorders of the bladder, genital apparatus and the rectum. The prostatic ducts are arranged in two groups around the urethra—an inner group of short ducts opening into the floor of the urethra and an outer group of longer ducts which open on either side of the verumontanum (*Fig.* 6.1). The prostatic arteries originate from the inferior vesical vessels and reach the gland on its infero-lateral aspect to run obliquely within the capsule and supply the fibro-muscular gland tissue and the prostatic urethra. A rich prostatic venous plexus drains into the internal iliac veins and lymphatic drainage is to the internal iliac and para-aortic lymph nodes.

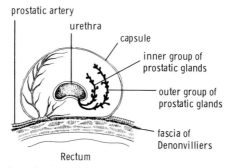

Fig. 6.1 Distribution of prostatic ducts and arteries at level of verumontanum.

The prostate gland is subject to hormonal influences throughout the male life span. In the intrauterine period the gland is stimulated by maternal oestrogens and oestrogenic activity may predominate in the latter decades of adult life. Androgenic stimulation of the prostate gland occurs during the active sexual period in the male—stimulation by the pituitary gland (interstitial-cell stimulating hormone) on the testes and thence on the prostate gland (*Fig.* 6.2). Prostatic gland secretion is important in spermatozoal activity and is rich in enzymic acid phosphatase. Serum prostatic acid phosphatase estimation (normal: 0–3 King-

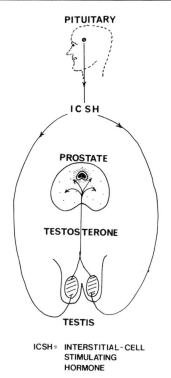

PITUITARY

IC SH

PROSTATE

TESTOSTERONE

TESTIS

ICSH = INTERSTITIAL-CELL
STIMULATING
HORMONE

Fig. 6.2. Hormonal stimulation of adult prostate gland.

–Armstrong units) is an indicator of glandular activity and the levels are frequently, though not invariably, elevated in patients with prostatic cancer.

• B. Inflammation of the Prostate Gland
Infection of the prostate gland may be acute or chronic.

Acute Prostatitis

Aetiology
1. Extension of gonococcal or non-specific urethritis.
2. Sequel of urethral instrumentation and catheterization.
3. Cystitis and upper tract infection.
4. Blood-borne infection.
5. Lymphatic permeation from rectum.
6. Organisms are usually *E. coli* or *S. faecalis*.

Clinical Features
Fever, rigors, dysuria, frequency, haematuria, retention of urine, perineal and

rectal pain (tenesmus). The inflamed gland is tense, swollen and tender and the patient may have an associated epididymo-orchitis.

Treatment
Bed rest, hot baths, analgesics, intramuscular or intravenous broad-spectrum antibiotics and suprapubic catheterization in patients with retention of urine.

Clinical Course of Prostatitis
A rapid response is achieved in most patients on systemic antibiotic therapy. Rarely, a prostatic abscess develops—diagnosed by feeling a boggy, fluctuant mass on rectal examination. The abscess always discharges per urethram with resolution of symptoms. Chronic prostatitis is a sequel of a prostatic abscess and will also develop in one third of patients with acute prostatitis (*Fig.* 6.3).

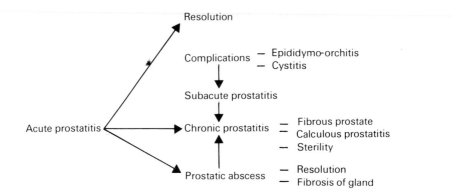

Fig. 6.3 Summary of pathological results of prostatic infection. *Note:* Tuberculous prostatitis is a manifestation of generalized genito-urinary tuberculosis.

Chronic Prostatitis
This condition may arise *de novo* via a blood-borne infection or as a sequel to acute inflammation of the gland or a prostatic abscess. The condition has a multiplicity of symptoms—generalized lethargy and ill-health, frequent, painful and difficult micturition, bouts of haematuria, perineal pain and aching, haemospermia, epididymitis and impotence. The prostate gland is hard and feels fibrotic on rectal examination (fibrous prostate). Relapses of infection are common and prostatic calculi and posterior urethral strictures will develop in most patients. The condition is extremely difficult to treat and eradicate—relapses are treated by antibiotic therapy and obstructive symptoms by perurethral resection.

Prostatic Calculi
Prostatic calculi form in the acini of the prostate gland—
1.   Associated with chronic prostatitis.
2.   Seen radiologically in region of symphysis pubis (*Fig.* 6.4).
3.   Black in colour and seen endoscopically in the ducts around the verumontanum.

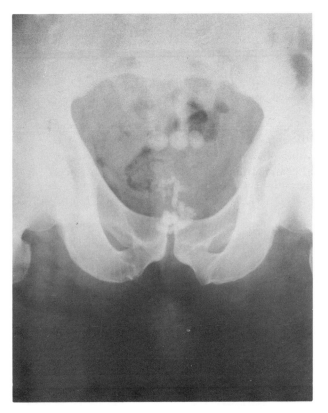

Fig. 6.4 Radiograph of bladder area showing prostatic calcification and three bladder stones.

4. Large number of calculi (calculous prostatitis) in the gland produce egg-shell crepitus on rectal examination.
5. No treatment indicated for calculi *per se* but may be indicated for co-existing chronic prostatitis.

- ### C. Bladder Outflow Obstruction: Benign Prostatic Hypertrophy

Bladder Outflow Obstruction

Mechanical and functional obstruction to the bladder outlet occurs either as a congenital condition or as an acquired problem later in life:

1. Congenital:
    Bladder outlet stenosis.
2. Acquired:
    Adult bladder neck obstruction (Marion's disease).

Fibrous prostate.
Benign prostatic hypertrophy (prostatomegaly).
Carcinoma of prostate gland.

Congenital Bladder Outlet Stenosis
A rare condition of infancy and childhood.
Diagnosis
Evidence of:
Clinically palpable non-tender bladder.
Endoscopic hypertrophy and trabeculation of the bladder with a normal bladder outlet.
Radiologically—upper tract dilatation.
Exclusion of:
Neurogenic bladder lesion.
Other causes of urethral obstruction.
Treatment
Endoscopic incision of bladder neck (*Fig.* 6.5), or Y–V-plasty of bladder neck (*Fig.* 6.6).

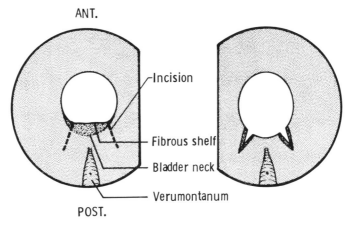

Fig. 6.5 Endoscopic incision of bladder neck.

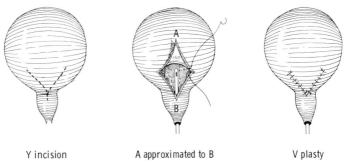

Fig. 6.6 Y–V-plasty of bladder neck.

Adult Bladder Neck Obstruction
A rare condition.
Suggested Aetiology
Dysrhythmia between the detrusor muscle and bladder neck sphincters.
Clinical Features and Diagnosis
1. Young patient.
2. Normal prostate gland.
3. No neurogenic bladder lesion.
4. IVU:
    Residual urine.
    Upper tract dilatation in 10 per cent.
5. Urinary flow rate:
    Grossly retarded with history of lifelong difficulty in passing urine.
6. Video-cystometry:
    Bladder neck dysrhythmia.
7. Cystoscopy:
    Normal prostate and prostatic urethra. Fibrous shelf (Marion) at posterior rim of bladder neck.

Treatment
No surgical treatment is necessary in most patients, but obstruction to upper tract and severe symptoms (10 per cent) may require bladder neck incision (*Fig.* 6.5).
Note:
    Complication after bladder neck incision—retrograde ejaculation will occur in 25–50 per cent of cases. Bladder neck incision must be advised with care for young males wishing to father children.

Benign Prostatic Hypertrophy

Incidence
1. Hypertrophy of the prostate gland occurs in 40 per cent of white males over 50 years of age.
2. 12 per cent of males over 70 years will require a prostatectomy.
3. Common in Western white races.
4. Relatively rare in Indian males.
5. Extremely rare in Negroes.

Aetiology
Unknown: related to hormonal changes in the male with advance in years: increased oestrogenic stimulation with concomitant decline in androgenic activity (the male menopause).

Pathology
Hypertrophy commences in the inner zone of prostatic glands (*Fig.* 6.7). Progressive enlargement compresses the outer zone of prostate gland to form a false capsule, indenting and distorting the prostatic urethra. The arterial blood supply to the prostate gland lies in the true capsule and the plane between true and false capsules is relatively avascular. Enlargement usually involves the lateral prostatic lobes but occasionally only the middle lobe is involved. The middle lobe is the portion of gland lying between the prostatic utricle and base of the bladder (*Fig.*

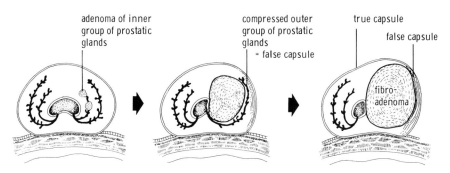

Fig. 6.7 Hypertrophy of prostate from inner zone of prostatic glands.

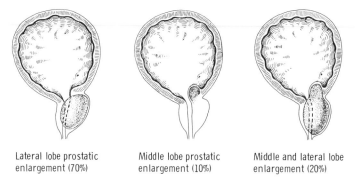

Lateral lobe prostatic enlargement (70%)

Middle lobe prostatic enlargement (10%)

Middle and lateral lobe enlargement (20%)

Fig. 6.8 Main categories of prostatic hypertrophy.

6.8). The enlarged middle lobe can act as a ball-valve and obstruct the bladder outlet. Histologically, the hypertrophied prostate consists of prostatic glands (adenosis), precursor cells for the glands (epitheliosis) and fibrous tissue (fibrosis).

Effects of Prostatic Enlargement (*Fig.* 6.9)
1.   On the urethra—elongation, compression, distortion, obstruction.
2.   On the bladder—hypertrophy, trabeculation, sacculation, diverticulae.
3.   On the ureters—elevation of the trigone, ureteric reflux, hydroureter.
4.   On the kidneys—hydronephrosis, chronic renal failure.

Secondary Effects
1.   Residual urine.
2.   Infection—prostatitis, cystitis, pyelonephritis.
3.   Stone formation.
4.   Possible bladder tumour due to urinary stasis.
5.   Acute or chronic retention of urine.

Clinical Features
A patient suffering from benign prostatic hypertrophy will be symptomless or will present with prostatism, acute or chronic retention of urine.

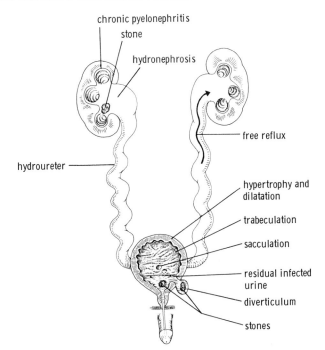

Fig. 6.9 Pathological changes in urinary tract in advanced obstructive uropathy.

1.   Prostatism:
          Delay in starting micturition.
          Poor stream.
          Dribbling and terminal incontinence.
          Frequency and nocturia.
          Feeling of incomplete emptying of bladder.
          Rectal pressure from enlargement of prostate—haemorrhoids.
          Straining to micturate—inguinal herniae.
2.   Acute retention:
          Sudden painful stoppage of urine.
          40 per cent—no prostatism.
          60 per cent—history of prostatism.
          Congestive cardiac failure.
          Drugs—atropine, pro-banthine, tricyclic antidepressants.
          Suppression of micturition.
          Alcoholic excesses.
          After instrumentation of the urethra.
3.   Chronic retention:
          Slow, progressive bladder outlet obstruction with overflow of urine.
          Distended painless, palpable bladder.
          Increase in abdominal girth.
          Rectal pressure and haemorrhoids.
          Bilateral direct herniae.
          Stigmata of chronic renal failure—uraemia, anaemia.

Note:

In 50 per cent of patients chronic retention of urine is caused by a middle lobe enlargement of the prostate gland.

Clinical Examination
General examination should include:
1. Elderly age group—cardiovascular and pulmonary assessment.
2. Conjunctivae, nail beds and palms—anaemia.
3. Tongue—furred and uraemic smell.
4. Abdominal palpation—renal enlargement, bladder distension.
5. Rectal examination:
    Firm elastic enlargement of lateral lobes: presence of median sulcus between lobes: movement of rectal mucosa over enlarged gland.

Diagnosis and Investigations
Acute and chronic retention of urine can be clinically diagnosed—palpable and percussible bladder. Benign hypertrophy of the prostate gland is diagnosed by a rectal examination.
1. Haemoglobin and white cell count:
    Anaemia and systemic infection.
2. Urinalysis and urinary culture:
    Urinary infection.
3. Prostatic acid phosphatase:
    Exclude prostatic carcinoma.
4. Serum electrolyte estimation:
    Raised urea and creatinine in renal failure.
5. IVU:
    Prostatic impression in cystogram phase (*Fig*. 6.10) with post-micturition residual urine: thickening of bladder wall and evidence of upper tract obstruction.
6. Ultrasonography:
    Full bladder examination—thickening of bladder wall and intravesical projection of prostate.
7. Cystourethroscopy:
    Trabeculation, sacculation, diverticulae, stones, infection and accurate bimanual assessment of size of hypertrophied prostate gland.
    Appearance of bladder neck (*Fig*. 6.11).

Management of Patients with Prostatism
1. Discovery of a large symptomless prostate gland on rectal examination—not an indication for operation.
2. Prostatism—complications (obstruction, stones, diverticulae)—prostatectomy. In this group troublesome nocturia (three or four times a night), wetting of underclothes or bed linen and attacks of near-acute retention of urine are indications for operation. The patient's age is irrelevant provided he is reasonably fit and can withstand a general or spinal anaesthetic.
3. Poor risk patients with severe prostatism—home catheter drainage for three or four months and physical reassessment at the end of this period.

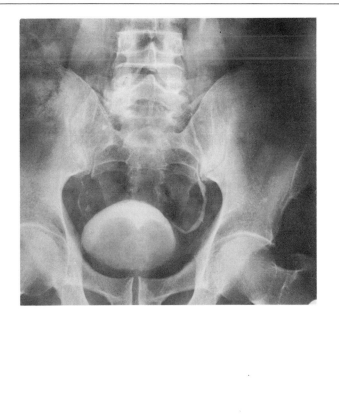

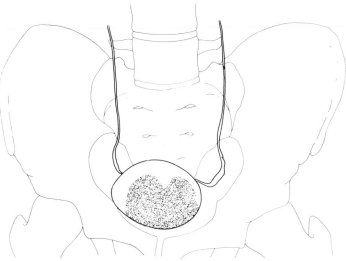

Fig. 6.10 IVU—impression in base of bladder due to hypertrophy of prostate gland.

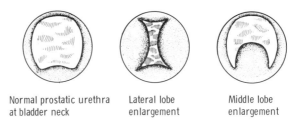

Normal prostatic urethra Lateral lobe Middle lobe
at bladder neck enlargement enlargement

Fig. 6.11 Endoscopic appearances of bladder neck in prostatic hypertrophy.

Management of Acute Retention of Urine
Urgent hospital admission is required, with:
1. Catheterization with sterile precautions.
2. Antibiotic therapy.
3. Emergency IVU.
4. General physical examination.
5. Prostatectomy within four days of admission.

If patient is unfit for operation or in the presence of urinary infection, continue catheter drainage for 7–20 days prior to prostatectomy. At the end of three weeks, if the patient's condition will still not allow an operation, he is sent home on catheter drainage to be readmitted in three months for reassessment and prostatectomy. Ninety per cent of patients admitted with acute retention of urine will be suitable for operation within three or four days of admission.

Management of Chronic Retention of Urine
Semi-urgent hospital admission, with the following treatment:
1. Bladder not catheterized.
2. Urgent biochemical investigation for renal failure.
3. Antibiotic therapy to prevent infection.
4. IVU and isotope renography not helpful.
5. General physical assessment and correction of anaemia.
6. Fit patient with satisfactory renal function (urea <11 mmol/l)—one-stage prostatectomy.
7. Unfit patient or impaired renal function (urea >11 mmol/l)—suprapubic catheter drainage for a few weeks to many months to allow recovery of renal function prior to elective prostatectomy. Sixty per cent of patients admitted with chronic retention of urine will be suitable for elective prostatectomy within 10 days of admission to hospital.

● **D. Prostatectomy**

Approaches to the Prostate Gland (*Fig.* 6.12)
1. Transvesical.
2. Retropubic.

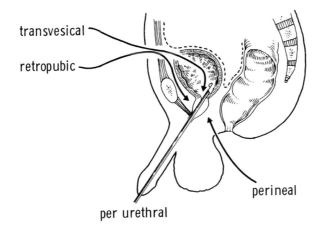

Fig. 6.12 Surgical approaches to the prostate gland.

3.   Perurethral.
4.   Perineal.
    A perineal approach to the prostate gland is rarely used in Britain but is popular in some centres in America. In the transvesical and retropubic operations the approach through the abdominal wall is similar, but in the transvesical procedure the bladder is opened (cystotomy), whilst in the retropubic operation the front of the prostatic capsule is incised. When the prostatic adenoma is enucleated the surgeon takes advantage of the relatively avascular plane between the true and false capsules of the prostate gland (*Fig*. 6.13).

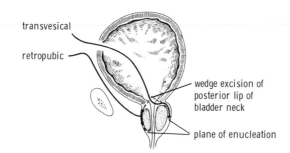

Fig. 6.13 Avascular plane of enucleation between true and false capsules in the transvesical and retropubic operations.

Choice of Operation
    A cystourethroscopy is mandatory in all patients as a preliminary examination to exclude bladder tumours or stones.
1.   Large glands (clinically estimated > 50 g)—retropubic prostatectomy.
2.   Smaller glands (clinically estimated < 50 g)—perurethral resection (*Fig*. 6.14).
3.   A transvesical prostatectomy is preferred to the retropubic operation in

obese patients, in infection of the retropubic space and in patients with hip deformities.

4.   In British hospital practice:

   60 per cent of operations are perurethral resections.
   30 per cent of operations are retropubic.
   10 per cent of operations are transvesical.

Perurethral Resection

The technique entails the use of a cutting diathermy loop (*Fig.* 6.14) for resection of segments of the hypertrophied prostate. It is the operation of choice for hypertrophied glands of small size (< 50 g), for middle lobe and bladder neck hypertrophy and for resection of a prostatic carcinoma. Complications of perurethral resection include:

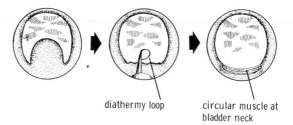

diathermy loop   circular muscle at
                     bladder neck

Fig. 6.14 Perurethral resection of hypertrophied middle lobe of prostate gland.

1.   Possible perforation of the bladder.
2.   Postoperative stricture of the prostatic urethra.
3.   Postoperative incontinence—damage to the sphincter muscles.
4.   Recurrent pathology—inadequate resection.

The disadvantages are minimized by increasing expertise of the operating surgeon.

Postoperative Management after Prostatectomy

1.   Indwelling Foley three-way catheter with continuous irrigation and drainage for 4–5 days.
2.   Maintenance of blood volume by adequate transfusion for blood loss.
3.   Antibiotic therapy in the presence of urinary infection.
4.   Large fluid intake and intravenous fluids for the first 48 hr.
5.   Early ambulation and physiotherapy for the chest and lower limbs.

Complications of Prostatectomy

1.   Immediate (within 48 hr):
   Primary (reactionary) haemorrhage.
   Bladder perforation (in perurethral resection).
   Cardiovascular and cerebral accidents.
2.   Intermediate (within 10 days):
   Secondary haemorrhage.
   Infection.
   Pulmonary infection, atelectasis and embolism.

Vascular:
  Myocardial infarct.
  Cerebral thrombosis.
3.   Remote (after 1 month):
  Incontinence.
  Urethral stricture.
  'Osteitis pubis'.

Management of Complications of Prostatectomy
1.   Primary and secondary arterial haemorrhage:
  Re-operation and ligation or endoscopic diathermy of bleeding vessel.
2.   Infection:
  Adequate antibiotic therapy.
3.   Perforation:
  Re-operation and closure of perforation.
4.   Embolism:
  Anticoagulant therapy.
5.   Stricture:
  Posterior urethra (infection)—dilatation and internal urethrotomy.
  Anterior urethra (instrumental trauma or damage by catheter)—dilatation and anterior urethroplasty.
6.   Incontinence (damage to sphincter):
  Incontinent appliances or penile clips: insertion of electrically controlled artificial sphincter in selected cases (p. 102).

Results of Prostatectomy
1.   Overall mortality:
  2 per cent—mainly from cardiac, cerebral and pulmonary complications.
2.   Morbidity:
  20 per cent—stricture: urinary incontinence.
  Satisfactory outcome after prostatectomy in 80 per cent of patients.

● **E. Carcinoma of the Prostate Gland**

Incidence
1.   Britain—fourth commonest malignant tumour in man following bronchogenic, colorectal and gastric tumours. Tumour is on the increase: 6000 new cases present each year. Second commonest malignant tumour of the genito-urinary tract after bladder carcinoma.
2.   Five per cent incidence in operative specimens for benign hypertrophy of the prostate.
3.   Scandinavia—high incidence.
4.   Far East—low incidence.

5.   USA:
        Second commonest malignant tumour following bronchogenic
        carcinoma.
        Higher incidence in Black Americans than in Caucasians.

Aetiology
        Persistent androgenic activity in males beyond the point of normal decline
(around 55 years of age) may contribute to continued stimulation of the prostatic
cells and neoplastic change. Most prostatic tumours are hormone dependent and
are controlled to a greater or lesser degree by oestrogen therapy or castration, a
concept introduced by Professor Charles Huggins of Chicago in 1941.

Pathology
1.   Carcinoma of the prostate occurs in 50–80 age group.
2.   80 per cent of the tumours become evident between 60 and 80 years of age.
3.   10 per cent of hospital admissions for retention of urine are due to a
        prostatic cancer.
4.   95 per cent of prostatic tumours are adenocarcinomas.
5.   The tumour starts in the epithelial cells of the ducts and acini in the outer
        zone of prostatic ducts (*Fig.* 6.15).
6.   20 per cent—multifocal tumours.

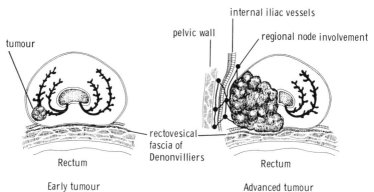

Fig. 6.15 Pathology of prostatic carcinoma.

Spread of Prostatic Carcinoma
1.   Local:
        Capsule of the prostate, trigone, seminal vesicles, lower end of
        ureters, prostatic urethra and para-rectal tissues. Spread into the
        rectal wall is limited by the rectovesical fascia of Denonvilliers.
2.   Lymphatic:
        Internal and common iliac nodes and late spread to the para-aortic
        nodes.
3.   Blood-borne:
        Bones—osteosclerotic deposits in the pelvic girdle, lumbar spine,
        femora and ribs in decreasing order of incidence (*Fig.* 6.16).

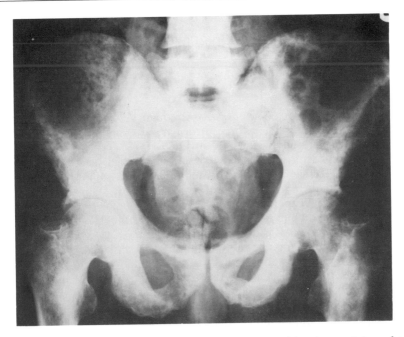

Fig. 6.16 Sclerotic metastases in pelvic bones and lumbar vertebrae from a primary prostatic carcinoma.

Lungs—pulmonary metastases are present in 25 per cent of patients with terminal prostatic cancer.

TNM Staging of Tumour

Combination of digital rectal examination, ultrasound, lymphography, bone scan and histology.

1. T: Tumour:
   - TIS—carcinoma in situ.
   - T0—incidental histological finding in a prostatectomy specimen.
   - T1—tumour within capsule surrounded by normal gland.
   - T2—tumour involving capsule—obliteration of median sulcus.
   - T3—extracapsular spread.
   - T4—tumour fixed and infiltrating neighbouring structures.
2. N: Nodes—not clinically assessable—demonstrated by lymphography and at operation:
   - N0—regional nodes not involved.
   - N1—single regional node involved.
   - N2—multiple regional nodes involved.
   - N3—fixed regional nodes in lateral pelvic wall.
   - N4—distant lymph nodes involved.
3. M: Metastases:
   - M0—no metastases.
   - M1—distant metastases—usually bones or lungs.

Histological Grading of Tumour
1. G1—highly differentiated—good prognosis.
2. G2—medium degree of differentiation.
3. G3—poorly differentiated.

Clinical Features
1. Local symptoms (77 per cent)—frequency, dysuria, haematuria, prostatism, dimunition in force of urinary stream, perineal pain, acute or chronic retention of urine.
2. Symptoms from metastases (16 per cent)—backache, sciatica, haemoptysis, swelling of legs due to femoral vein thrombosis. Erythroblastic anaemia due to replacement of bone marrow by malignant cells.
3. Asymptomatic patients (7 per cent)—incidental finding of a prostatic carcinoma on physical examination or histological examination of an excised or resected prostate gland.
4. Digital examination of the rectum provides a diagnosis in 75 per cent of patients. A prostatic carcinoma is rock hard, craggy or nodular on palpation and in T2 and T3 tumours the median sulcus between the lateral lobes is obliterated and the rectal mucosa 'fixed' to the gland. Advanced tumours (T3 and T4) will demonstrate lateral fixation to the sides of the bony pelvis and rectum.

Diagnosis and Investigation
1. Rectal examination.
2. Prostatic acid phosphatase estimation—in the normal prostate gland phosphatase acts as a catalyst for conversion of phosphate from the organic to the inorganic form and is active in an acid medium. Serum acid phosphatase is elevated in some patients with prostatic carcinoma, with gross elevation in some patients with bony metastases.
3. Ultrasound—determines size, position and extent of spread through the capsule of a prostatic tumour. The ultrasound probe is inserted into the rectum or urethra.

Radiology
1. Chest X-ray: Pulmonary metastases or rib deposits.
2. Lumbar spine and pelvis:
    Osteosclerotic metastases in vertebrae or pelvic bones (*Fig.* 6.16).
3. Bone scan:
    Sensitive indicator of early metastatic deposits (*Fig.* 6.17).
4. IVU:
    Bladder outlet obstruction, hydroureter and hydronephrosis.
5. Lymphography:
    Occasionally demonstrates involvement of internal iliac or para-aortic nodes (*Fig.* 6.18).

Operative
1. Cystourethroscopy:
    Visual evidence of obstructive uropathy.

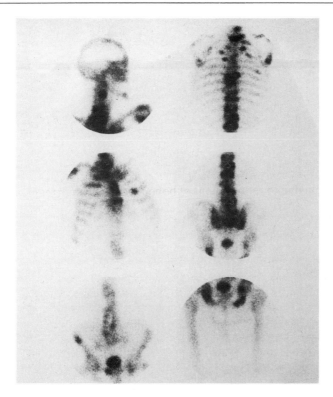

Fig. 6.17 Bone scan in prostatic carcinoma. 'Hot spots' due to metastatic deposits.

2.   Bimanual examination:
          Under anaesthesia: aid to accurate TNM staging of tumour.
3.   Biopsy:
          Positive confirmation of malignancy must be obtained in all patients before commencing treatment. A biopsy of the prostate may be obtained by one of four methods:
               Perurethral resection—therapeutic and relieves obstruction.
               Transvesical—at open operation on bladder and prostate gland.
               Transrectal needle biopsy.
               Perineal—percutaneous needle biopsy.

Treatment
          The policy for treatment of a prostatic carcinoma is governed by—
1.   The patient's age and general condition.
2.   TNM staging of the tumour.
3.   Histological grading of the tumour:
          TIS and T1 tumours diagnosed incidentally (7 per cent)—no treatment.
          T1 tumours with no symptoms or metastases—no treatment.

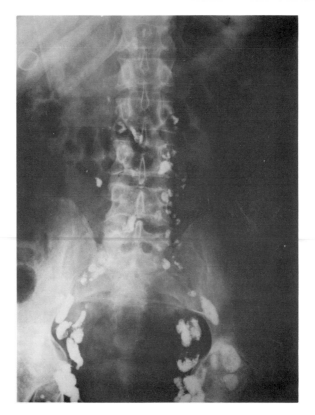

Fig. 6.18 Lymphogram. Left internal iliac node deposits in carcinoma of the prostate.

T1 tumours (symptomatic) but no metastases:
　　Perurethral resection.
　　Young patients + radiotherapy.
　　Old patients + hormone therapy or castration.
T2 tumours with or without metastases:
　　Perurethral resection combined with hormone therapy or
　　subcapsular orchidectomy (*Fig.* 6.19).

Incision of tunica
albuginea

Delivery and excision
of seminiferous tubules

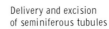
Resuturing of tunica
albuginea

Fig. 6.19 Subcapsular orchidectomy.

T3 and T4 tumours with or without metastases:
    Mega-voltage radiotherapy with hormone therapy or castration. Treatment is palliative.
All patients with bony metastases:
    Treated by either hormone therapy or subcapsular orchidectomy (castration). Local radiotherapy treatment for painful bony metastases.

Chemotherapeutic agents have proved disappointing in the management of advanced (T3, T4) prostatic cancer. These agents may have a palliative role in management when conventional treatment, hormone therapy or castration has failed in controlling the patient's symptoms.

Surgery in Management of Prostatic Carcinoma
It will be evident that perurethral resection is an important operation in the management of prostatic cancer and it operates both as a diagnostic and therapeutic measure. The role of total prostatectomy is debatable. This operation is popular in North America for T1 and T2 tumours but the operative results in terms of persistent fistulae, incontinence and stricture formation are often disappointing. The operation of total prostatectomy is rarely used in Great Britain in the management of prostatic cancer.

Medical Management of Prostatic Carcinoma

Hormone Therapy
Oestrogen (stilboestrol) has been used for decades in the management of prostatic carcinoma. The hormone has many undesirable side-effects, including congestive cardiac failure, cerebrovascular accidents, gynaecomastia and impotence. Severe side-effects will necessitate discontinuing the hormone in many cases.

Carcino-chemotherapeutic Drugs
Tetrasodium fosfestrol (Honvan) and estramustine phosphate (Estracyt)—combinations of hormone and chemotherapeutic agents—have fewer side-effects and are more commonly used in the medical management of prostatic carcinoma patients.

Present Advances in Treatment
Cyproterone acetate (Cyprostat) acts directly on the malignant tumour cells and is claimed specifically to retard extra-prostatic sites of androgen production.

Zoladex is an LH–RH analogue and appears to act centrally on the pituitary gland and hypothalamus, blocking stimulation by the pituitary in producing interstitial cell stimulating hormone (ICSH) and consequently the androgenic activity of the testes and adrenals (*Fig. 6.2*).

Prognosis
Suppression of androgenic activity of the prostate in patients with a carcinoma has a palliative effect on the patient's symptoms in most cases. Symptomatic relief is achieved in 75 per cent of patients and life expectancy of a prostatic cancer patient with a low grade tumour (G1, G2) is 5–7 years, despite the presence of bony metastatic disease.

Future Trends

These include:

1. Hormone assays on fresh specimens of prostatic cancer in an attempt to predict hormone dependability of the tumour and select the appropriate hormone for therapeutic use.

2. Percutaneous insertion of radioactive seeds into the prostate gland and tumour. For symptomatic T1 and T2 tumours radioactive iodine (I^{125}) seeds are inserted percutaneously through the perineum under ultrasound control for localized interstitial irradiation of the prostatic carcinoma.

7

The urethra

The Female Urethra
The female urethra is 3·3 cm in length. Its upper half is surrounded by the internal sphincter separated anteriorly from the pubovesical ligaments and symphysis pubis by fibro-fatty tissue and posteriorly partially embedded in the anterior wall of the vagina. The distal half below the urogenital diaphragm is surrounded by the external sphincter muscles and the urethral orifice is found in the anterior wall of the vaginal vestibule just posterior to the clitoris.

Congenital stenosis of the urethra may occur. The urethra may be injured in crush injuries of the pelvis. Most female urethral injuries are iatrogenic—inflicted by urological instruments and gynaecological repair procedures or self-inflicted by the patient herself during mechanical attempts at sexual excitation. Urethritis is nearly always the result of ascending infection from the vagina. It is a common symptom in venereal infection and frequently the presenting symptom of gonorrhoea in the female.

The Male Urethra

● A. Congenital Anomalies
1. Urethral valves.
2. Hypospadias.
3. Epispadias.

Posterior Urethral Valves
Posterior urethral valves are duplications of the urothelium in the region of the verumontanum, concave towards the bladder and obstructing urinary outflow but allowing easy passage of a catheter into the bladder. The valves form in early intra-uterine life and produce gross dilatation of the prostatic urethra, distension of the bladder, hydroureter and hydronephrosis (*Fig.* 7.1). Extreme cases (70 per cent) present at birth with a palpable bladder, ureters and kidneys, palpable

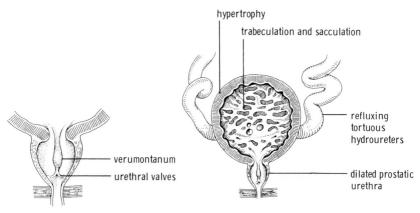

Fig. 7.1 Pathology of posterior urethral valves.

distension of the prostatic urethra on rectal examination, and severe renal impairment, often incompatible with survival. Milder cases may survive until childhood but will always have difficulty with micturition and a poor stream. Diagnosis is made by compression cystography (*Fig.* 7.2) and cystourethroscopy.

Treatment
Preliminary nephrostomy drainage in patients with hydronephrosis and hydroureter in renal failure. Endoscopic division of the valves or urinary diversion in end-stage renal disease.

Prognosis
Prognosis is poor—50 per cent of the infantile group only survive a few months.

Anterior Urethral Valves
These are very rare and present in childhood or young adult patients with a very poor urinary stream and a palpable bladder. Urethrography and cystourethroscopy will demonstrate distension of the anterior urethra behind the valves. Treatment is by endoscopic division of the valves and prognosis is excellent.

Hypospadias
Hypospadias is due to failure in development of the terminal urethra. The site of the urethral opening on the ventral surface of the penis may be glandular, coronal, penile, scrotal or perineal. Associated anomalies are:
1.   Meatal stenosis.
2.   Hooded foreskin.
3.   Chordee:
         Fibrosis along the line of the absent urethra, producing angulation of the penis (*Fig.* 7.3).

Incidence
1.   1 in 250 male infants.
2.   Familial history.

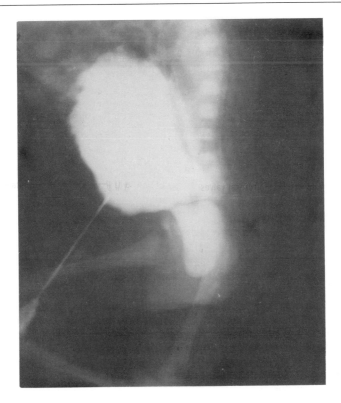

Fig. 7.2 Suprapubic cystography. Gross dilatation of prostatic urethra in urethral valves.

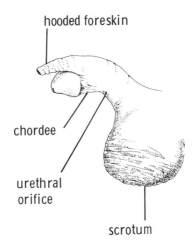

Fig. 7.3 Anomalies in penile hypospadias.

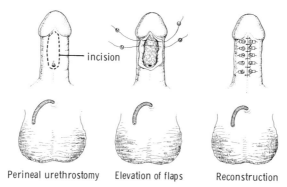

Perineal urethrostomy   Elevation of flaps   Reconstruction

Fig. 7.4 Denis–Browne method of hypospadias reconstruction.

Associated Anomalies

Maldescent of the testes and urinary tract anomalies are present in 20 per cent of patients.

Treratment

Definitive surgical treatmentent and a repair of the hypospadias (*Fig.* 7.4) are undertaken at four to five years of age before the boy attends primary school.

Meatal stenosis and chordee are corrected at 18 months. Correction of chordee allows elongation and growth of the penis. The hooded foreskin is not excised until a satisfactory repair has been attained: it may be used as a skin pedicle to cover the ventral orifice of the penis at a later operation.

Complications

1.   Urethral fistulae.
2.   Stenosis of the urethral repair.
3.   Growth of hair inside the reconstructed urethra.

Results of Repair Operations

The cosmetic and functional results of hypospadias repair are usually good but many operations may be necssary to achieve satisfaction.

Epispadias

Extremely rare anomaly. The urethral opening is on the dorsum of the penis and the penile shaft is grossly angulated. Severe forms of epispadias are associated with abnormality of the bladder sphincters and exstrophy of the bladder (p. 87).

● B. Urethral Trauma

Urethral injuries may be direct or indirect. The long-term sequelae of urethral damage are stricture formation, impotence and incontinence. Surgical treatment of urethral injuries is directed towards the prevention of these sequelae.

Direct trauma is iatrogenic and may occur during surgical instrumentation or be self-induced by the patient who attempts to negotiate his own urethra with various objects. The anterior urethra is sometimes injured by forcible bending of the erect penis (fracture of the penis).

Indirect trauma, due to an external force, may damage the bulbar or membranous urethra (*Fig. 7.5*).

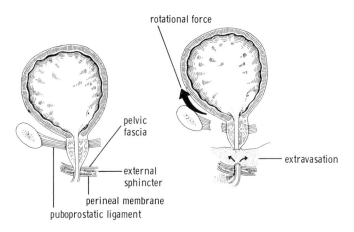

Fig. 7.5 Intrapelvic rupture of male urethra.

Urethral trauma may be classified as:
1.   Anterior:
        Iatrogenic—95 per cent.
        External trauma—5 per cent.
2.   Posterior:
        Bulbar:
                Iatrogenic—90 per cent.
                Astride injury—10 per cent.
        Membranous:
                Iatrogenic—70 per cent.
                Pelvic fracture—30 per cent.

Note:
    10 per cent of pelvic girdle fractures have a ruptured membranous urethra.

Anterior Urethral Injuries

Anterior urethral injuries present with a history of trauma, excessive swelling and bruising of the penis and bloody discharge from the external meatus.

Treatment

Suprapubic catheterization and gentle dilatation plus insertion of a soft urethral catheter after 7–10 days.

Bulbar Urethral Injuries

Commonest iatrogenic injury treated by urethral catheterization for 7–10 days. Rarer bulbar injury due to external trauma and crushing of the urethra against undersurface of pubic symphysis produces urethral bleeding and bruising of the perineum, scrotum, penis and lower abdominal wall. Attempts at micturition lead to extravasation of urine and increase in size of the perineo-scrotal swelling.

Management

Drainage of a large haematoma or of extravasated urine and suprapubic catheterization. Removal of the catheter after 10 days and careful observation during the ensuing months and years for development of a urethral stricture—flow rate studies, urethrography and urethroscopy.

Membranous Urethral Injury

The membranous urethra is 1–1·5 cm in length and lies within the pelvic cavity between the pelvic fascia superiorly and the perineal membrane inferiorly, surrounded by the external urethral sphincter (*Fig.* 1.4). The urethra at the perineal membrane is a fixed point and held in position by the pubo-vesical and pubo-urethral ligaments. A shearing force which disrupts the pelvic ring and separates the pubis from ischial rami may rupture the membranous urethra.

Diagnosis

Radiological evidence of a pelvic fracture, urethral bleeding, urine not voided since injury, a palpable distended bladder, upward displacement of the prostate gland on rectal examination.

Management

General resuscitation and urgent treatment for associated injuries. Attempt gentle urethral catheterization—if unsuccessful, suprapubic catheterization. In a membranous urethral rupture the aims of treatment are:
1. Diversion of urine from the site of rupture by suprapubic catheterization.
2. Alignment of the two urethral ends.
3. Maintenance of position of the aligned ends of the ruptured urethra.
4. Drainage of retropubic space—blood and extravasated urine.

Partial Rupture

Suprapubic exploration and catheterization plus 'rail-roading' of a catheter through the stricture from above and below (*Fig.* 7.6): drainage of retropubic space.

Complete Rupture

Suprapubic exploration and catheterization: introduction of catheter into bladder via the urethra to act as a splint: fixation of the apex of the prostate to the pelvic floor and drainage of the retropubic space.

Sequelae of Rupture of Membranous Urethra:
1. Incontinence—appears early—damage to urethral sphincters.
2. Impotence—appears early—severance of pelvic nerve plexuses.
3. Stricture—appears late—fibrosis.

Postoperative Management

Careful observation for years. Regular urinary flow rate estimation, urethrography and urethroscopy.

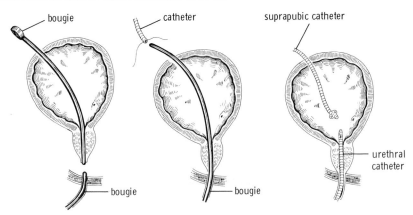

Contact between metal bougies

Fig. 7.6 'Rail-roading' method of alignment in partial urethral rupture.

Note:

Most patients who suffer injury to the membranous urethra will develop a urethral stricture, weeks, months or years after the original treatment.

●   **C. Urethral Infection**

Urethral infection is acute or chronic.

Acute Urethritis

1.   Venereal:

Gonorrhoea.

Syphilis.

Lympho-granuloma venereum.

Protozoal:

Trichomonas vaginalis.

Candida albicans.

2.   Non-venereal:

Mechanical trauma or foreign bodies.

Chemical or thermal burns.

Infection from prostate or bladder, perineum and penis.

Drug-induced (i.e. cantharides and phenolphthalein).

Non-specific urethritis.

Symptoms

1.   Scalding micturition.

2.   Urethral discharge.

3.   Soreness and itching of lips of external meatus.

Diagnosis

Microscopic examination and culture of urine and of urethral discharge.

Treatment
Bed rest, liberal fluid intake, appropriate antibiotics.
Note:
> Relapses of acute urethritis are common especially in patients with non-specific urethritis.

Complications
1. Chronic urethritis (relapsing).
2. Infection of periurethral glands—abscess or stricture.
3. Calculus formation.
4. Prostatitis.
5. Epididymo-orchitis.
6. Cystitis and acute pyelonephritis.
7. Urethritis with arthritis and conjunctivitis—Reiter's syndrome.

Peri-urethral Abscess
Infection in an obstructed para-urethral gland or proximal to an established urethral stricture. Developing abscess forms a tender mass along the under-surface of the penis with gross inflammatory oedema of the scrotum, penis and perineum. The abscess discharges into the urethra or externally to form a urethreal fistula, which may be multiple (gun-shot perineum) in venereal and tuberculous cases.

Immediate Treatment
Antibiotics and external drainage with suprapubic catheterization if the patient has acute retention of urine.

Later Treatment
Urethral dilatation and excision of fistula. Multiple fistulae excised with reconstruction of anterior urethra (*Fig.* 7.9).

Urethral Calculi
May form within obstructed para-urethral glands: may lodge in the urethra *en route* to the exterior from the bladder: may form within a urethral diverticulum. Most calculi are removed endoscopically but some will require excision via the penile shaft or perineum.

Urethral Foreign Bodies
Majority introduced into the urethra for sexual experimentation in childhood and sexual perversion in adult life. Sometimes a catheter tip may be left in the urethra. Foreign bodies in the urethra are removed endoscopically via the external meatus.

• D. Urethral Strictures
A urethral stricture is a congenital or pathological narrowing of the urethral wall which will not allow functional dilatation of the urethra during

onward passage of urine. A stricture may be congenital, traumatic, inflammatory or neoplastic in origin.

1. Congenital:
     Pin-hole meatal stenosis.
     Associated with hypospadias or phimosis.
2. Traumatic:
     Instrumentation and perurethral resection.
     Operations on the bladder neck, prostate and urethra.
     Rupture of the urethra in pelvic injuries.
     Rarely in the female at childbirth.
     Note:
          Traumatic strictures involve a short segment of the urethra.
3. Inflammatory:
     Gonococcal, non-specific urethritis, tuberculosis.
     Prolonged catheterization.
     Note:
          Inflammatory strictures are long and often multiple.
4. Neoplastic:
     A tumour within the urethral wall or outside the urethra will produce narrowing and stricture formation.

Pathology

Slow progressive fibrosis produces secondary changes of chronic outflow obstruction with hypertrophy of the bladder, hydroureter and hydronephrosis in advanced cases (*Fig.* 7.7).

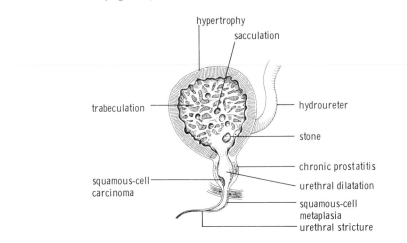

Fig. 7.7 Secondary pathological results of a urethral stricture.

Clinical Features

Presenting complaint—poor, thin, deviating stream, with terminal dribbling, frequency and scalding on micturition, if secondary infection is present. The bladder may be chronically distended. Strictures of the anterior urethra are sometimes palpable along the penile shaft.

Investigations
1. Urinary flow rate—diminished in stricture patients.
2. IVU—evidence of upper tract dilatation and post-micturition residual urine.
3. Urethrography—demonstrates the site, length and number of urethral strictures (*Fig.* 7.8).
4. Urethroscopy—direct visualization of urethral strictures.

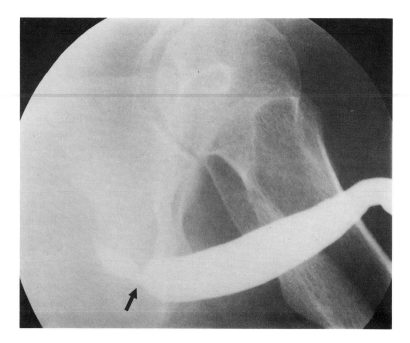

Fig. 7.8 Urethrography. Bulbar urethral stricture.

Management
There are three methods of management:
1. Dilatation.
2. Endoscopic division—internal urethrotomy.
3. Urethroplastic procedures.
Method selected will depend on patient's age, general condition, site, length and number of urethral strictures.
1. Elderly and infirm patients—repeated dilatation (three-monthly).
2. Younger fit age group:
    Operative treatment.
    Internal urethrotomy, i.e. endoscopic division of stricture under direct vision.
    Successful in 80 per cent of patients: may have to be repeated.

In 20 per cent of urethral strictures an open operation is necessary.
1. Anterior urethra—anterior urethroplasty (*Fig.* 7.9).
2. Posterior urethra—posterior scrotal (inlay) urethroplasty.

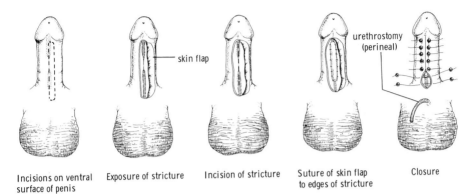

Incisions on ventral surface of penis | Exposure of stricture | Incision of stricture | Suture of skin flap to edges of stricture | Closure

Fig. 7.9 Excision and reconstruction of anterior urethral stricture.

Results of Urethroplasty
Poor results in majority of posterior urethral strictures, due to recurrent stricture formation.

• E. Urethral Tumours
Urethral tumours are very rare. In patients with a bladder carcinoma secondary tumours may be found in the urethra at routine cystourethroscopy—modified transitional cell carcinoma—treated by endoscopic resection and diathermy or a radical cystourethrectomy in continuity with the bladder tumour. Malignant tumours arising in association with a urethral stricture are usually squamous cell carcinomata—treated by external radiotherapy, penile amputation and, in the presence of lymph node metastases, block dissection of the groin.

8

Penis and scrotum

- ### A. Congenital Anomalies

The post-pubertal penis may be underdeveloped (micro-penis) and associated with poor testicular development (hypogonadism). A double penis (diphallus) is an extremely rare anomaly and associated with urethral duplication. The scrotum may develop in two separate sacs (bifid scrotum) and occasionally one half of the scrotum remains underdeveloped—associated with absence or maldescent of a testis on the corresponding side.

Phimosis

Phimosis—inablity to retract the foreskin.

Paraphimosis—inability to reduce a retracted foreskin.

The foreskin is normally adherent to the glans penis until the age of 2–3 years. Thereafter, inability to retract the foreskin indicates some degree of phimosis. Phimosis may be congenital or acquired:

1. Congenital phimosis—two types of foreskin are recognized in infants:
   The truncated foreskin—partially retractible to show the end of the glans penis—90 per cent.
   The phimotic foreskin—10 per cent—flattened over the end of the glans with a narrow, circular and rigid orifice (*Fig.* 8.1).
2. Acquired phimosis—found in older children and adults as the result of:
   Persistence of congenital phimosis.
   Recurrent infections (balanitis).
   Development of diabetes.
   Underlying tumour of the glans penis.

- ### B. Circumcision

Circumcision is an operation for removal of the foreskin.

Medical Indications for Circumcision

Infants

1. Religious ritual circumcision—Jews, Arabs and Muslims.
2. Persistence of congenital phimosis (10 per cent) with ballooning of foreskin.

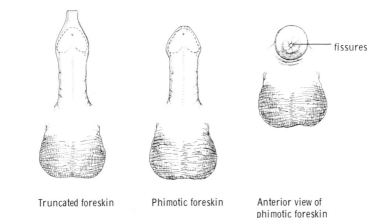

Truncated foreskin   Phimotic foreskin   Anterior view of
                                           phimotic foreskin

Fig. 8.1 Congenital anomalies of foreskin.

3.   Paraphimosis.
4.   Recurrent balanitis.
5.   Removal of hooded foreskin in hypospadias.

Adults
1.   Recurrent balanitis.
2.   Diabetes.
3.   Preputial injuries.
4.   Paraphimosis.
5.   Underlying tumour of the glans penis.

Social Indications for Operation
Few, if any, are pertinent, apart from the ritual group of patients. There is some evidence that circumcision reduces the incidence of penile carcinoma in the male and cervical carcinoma in the female.

Operation of Circumcision
There are three main techniques:
1.   Formal circumcision (*Fig.* 8.2).
2.   Crushing of foreskin with bone-cutting forceps.
3.   Plastibell operation (*Fig.* 8.3) for infants.

Complications of Operation
1.   Primary or secondary haemorrhage.
2.   Secondary infection—very common.
3.   Ulceration of unprotected glans—meatal stenosis.
4.   Too radical excision of the foreskin.
5.   Injury or excision of the glans.
6.   Death from anaesthesia or complication of circumcision.
       Circumcision must never be regarded as a 'minor op'. The operation must always be undertaken by a trained surgeon under general anaesthesia administered by an expert anaesthetist.

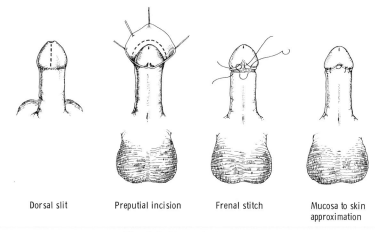

Dorsal slit Preputial incision Frenal stitch Mucosa to skin approximation

Fig. 8.2 Formal circumcision.

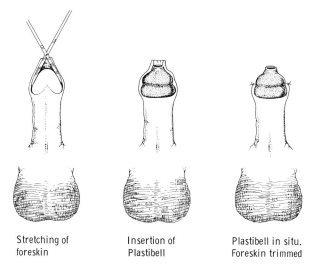

Stretching of foreskin Insertion of Plastibell Plastibell in situ. Foreskin trimmed

Fig. 8.3 Plastibell method of circumcision.

C. Miscellaneous Conditions of the Penis and Scrotum

Peyronie's Disease (Cavernositis)

This condition affects men between 40 and 60 years of age and causes deformity of the erect penis, interfering with intercourse, and occasionally producing impotence. The lesion is a fibrous or calcified plaque of tissue in the corpora cavernosa. Spontaneous resolution of the condition may occur after months or several years. There is no satisfactory treatment for Peyronie's cavernositis. Excision of the fibrous plaque usually results in further deformity of the penis.

Priapism

Priapism is defined as persistent painful erection. Possible causes are listed below:
1. Primary idiopathic (80 per cent).
2. Secondary (20 per cent).
   Leukaemia.
   Sickle cell anaemia.
   Ulcerative colitis.
   Disseminated malignant disease.
   Haemodialysis.

Note:
Priapism is occasionally the presenting symptom in patients who will subsequently develop leukaemia or ulcerative colitis.

Blood within the corpora cavernosa becomes thick and viscid. The priapism resolves in two or three weeks and the corpora are replaced by fibrous tissue. The patient is impotent.

Treatment—emergency procedure—anastomosis of the long saphenous vein to the distended corpora cavernosa, establishing venous drainage of the corpora.

Infective Gangrene of the Scrotum (Fournier's Gangrene)

Infection of scrotal skin with mixed organisms including anaerobic streptococci, producing scrotal gangrene and sloughing. Treatment—intensive antibiotic therapy, excision of areas of dead scrotal skin and skin grafting.

• D. Tumours of the Penis and Scrotum

Tumours of the penis are benign or malignant. The commonest benign tumour is a papilloma. Multiple papillomatous lesions are found on the glans penis and prepuce in venereal infection—condyloma acuminata. The commonest malignant penile tumour is a squamous cell carcinoma of the glans penis.

Carcinoma of the Penis

Incidence
1. Accounts for 1·25 per cent of all malignant tumours in male patients aged between 60 and 80 years.
2. A penile carcinoma does not occur in circumcized patients.
3. Phimosis of varying degree is present in 80 per cent of patients.
4. No carcinogenic agents have been isolated from adult smegma.

Pathology

The tumour commences in the sulcus between the glans penis and prepuce as an ulcerating or proliferative lesion which bleeds easily and becomes secondarily infected. Local spread tethers and contracts the foreskin—phimosis. Lymphatic spread is to the inguinal nodes, palpably enlarged in 70 per cent of patients (*Fig.* 8.4).

Inguinal lymphadenopathy:
50 per cent metastatic.
50 per cent infective.

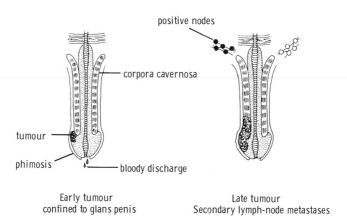

Early tumour
confined to glans penis
(Prognosis: - 90% 5 yr. cure)

Late tumour
Secondary lymph-node metastases
(Prognosis: - 38% 5 yr. cure)

Fig. 8.4 Pathology of carcinoma of glans penis.

Clinical Features

Offensive, bloody discharge with tethered foreskin or phimosis and a palpable lump beneath the foreskin. Inguinal lymphadenopathy in 70 per cent of patients—inflammatory nodes or secondary lymph node metastases.

Diagnosis

Biopsy, combined with a dorsal slit or circumcision in phimosis.

Treatment

1. Tumour confined to glans penis (T1 and T2)—external radiotherapy.
2. Large infective fungating tumour (T3)—partial or radical amputation of penis.
3. Inguinal lymphadenopathy—biopsy after primary treatment is complete.
4. Malignant lymph node deposits—regional block dissection (*Fig.* 8.5) or local radiotherapy.
5. Advanced tumours with involvement of internal iliac nodes—chemotherapy.

Prognosis

Radiotherapy and partial amputation for early T1 and T2 tumours—90 per cent 5-year survival.

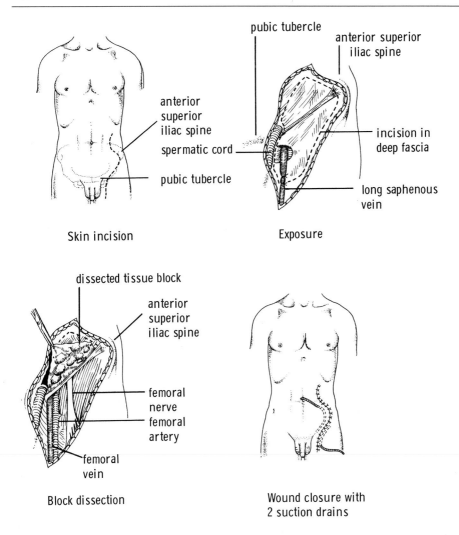

Skin incision

Exposure

Block dissection

Wound closure with
2 suction drains

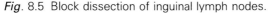

Fig. 8.5 Block dissection of inguinal lymph nodes.

Tumours of the Scrotum

The commonest benign scrotal 'tumour' is a sebaceous cyst.

Malignant tumours of the scrotum are squamous cell carcinoma. Historically these tumours occurred in chimney sweeps (chimney sweep cancer) and cotton spinners (mule-spinner's cancer), the irritant carcinogens in each group being soot and shale oil respectively. Treatment is by hemi-scrotectomy and orchidectomy, combined with an inguinal node block dissection on the affected side.

9

Testis, epididymis and spermatic cord

● **A. Congénital Anomalies of the Testis**

Maldescent of the Testes and the Ectopic Testis

The testes develop during the 5th week of intrauterine life from genital ridges on the posterior abdominal wall. A band of mesenchyme (eventually the gubernaculum) connects the developing testis to the inguinal region. Final descent of the testis occurs within the protrusion of peritoneum into the scrotum (processus vaginalis) during the last month of intrauterine life. The processus eventually becomes obliterated, leaving its distal end to surround the testes within the scrotum (the vaginal sac) (*Fig.* 9.1). In maldescent of the testis arrest occurs along this line of normal descent. In the ectopic testis the organ has deviated away from its normal line of descent and may lie in the inguinal area (superficial inguinal pouch), in front of the penis (prepenile), in the perineum or in the thigh (*Fig.* 9.2).

Incidence
1.　30 per cent of premature infants—maldescent of both testes.
2.　 3 per cent of full-term infants—maldescent at birth.
3.　 1 per cent of infants after 1 year—maldescent.
　　　Spontaneous descent after 1 year will probably not occur.

Clinical Features
An empty scrotal sac in a male child over 1 year of age indicates that the testes may be:
1.　Absent (4 per cent).
2.　Bilaterally absent (0·5 per cent).
3.　Retractile.
4.　Ectopic.
5.　Truly maldescended.
　　　The rectractile testis can be coaxed gently with warm hands into the scrotum, but will spring back into the inguinal region under the palpating fingers. Normal descent will occur and the parent and child are reassured. The ectopic testis may be palpable in the superficial inguinal pouch (*Fig.* 9.3), in front of the symphysis pubis or in the thigh and cannot be brought into the scrotum. The truly

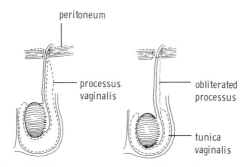

Fig. 9.1 Development of vaginal sac in scrotum.

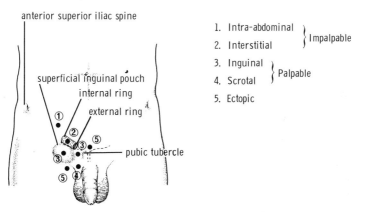

Fig. 9.2 Positions of maldescended and ectopic testis.

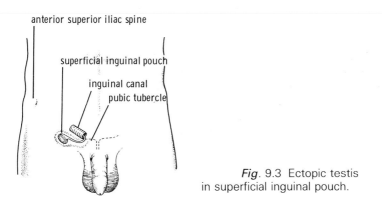

Fig. 9.3 Ectopic testis
in superficial inguinal pouch.

maldescended testis may be in the inguinal canal (impalpable), at the external ring or scrotal neck (palpable) but cannot be brought into the scrotum by digital manipulation. Operative treatment is indicated for the ectopic and maldescended testis after a diagnosis is established and before 4 years of age, so that the testis may be allowed to develop in its normal environment.

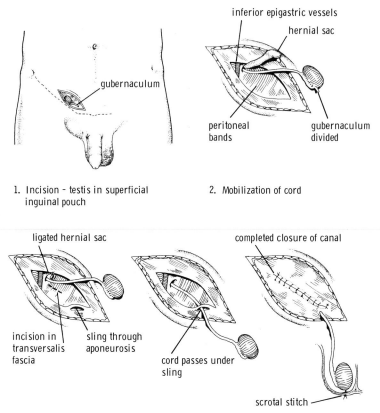

1. Incision - testis in superficial inguinal pouch

2. Mobilization of cord

3. Fixation of testis

Fig. 9.4 Denis-Browne method of orchidopexy.

Pathology and Complications

A maldescended testis will not develop normally and spermatogenesis is adversely affected. The conditions associated with maldescent of the testis are:

1. Infertility:

    Bilateral maldescent—patient nearly always infertile. Seminiferous tubules develop between 3 and 5 years of age. Essential that the testes should be in the scrotal sac by the age of 5 years.

2. Torsion:

    The maldescended testis is liable to undergo torsion.

3. Trauma:

    The maldescended testis is relatively fixed and exposed to injury from indirect trauma.

4. Hernia:

    Majority have an associated hernial sac.

5. Cosmetic:

    Older boys are often acutely concious of the anatomy of their external genitalia.

6.   Malignancy:
            1 in 1500 chance of developing a testicular tumour.
            40 times greater incidence of malignancy than in a normally
            descended testis.
            Correction of maldescent after puberty does not diminish the risk of
            malignant change.

Surgical Treatment
The aim of the surgeon in all patients with maldescended or ectopic testes is to
bring the organs with their blood supply into the scrotum without tension by the
age of 4 years.
1.   Age of presentation 3–4 years—orchidopexy.
2.   Age of presentation 5–12 years:
            Well-developed testis—orchidopexy.
            Poorly developed testis—orchidectomy.
3.   Presentation after 12 years:
            Well-developed testis (rare)—orchidopexy.
            Poorly developed testis—orchidectomy (*Fig.* 9.14).
Note:
        Hormone therapy is not usually of any benefit in the management of a
        maldescended testis.
Orchidopexy
The essential points in the operative technique are full mobilization of the cord
to the internal ring, excision of the associated hernial sac, placement and fixation
of the vascular testis in the scrotum without tension on the cord or testicular
vessels (*Fig.* 9.4).

• B. Trauma and Torsion of the Testis

Trauma
        Direct injury to the testis may occur in road traffic and industrial
accidents. The scrotum is often lacerated and the testis prolapses through the
disrupted scrotal skin. Damage to the tunica albuginea of the testis allows the
seminiferous tubules to prolapse through the laceration (hernia testis). Treatment is conservative whenever possible; an orchidectomy is indicated for gross
damage to the testis.

Torsion of the Testis
        Twisting of the testis on the spermatic cord interferes with its blood
supply and if untreated leads to gangrene. Torsion of the testis occurs in the
neonatal period or at puberty and early adulthood.
        In neonatal torsion, the infant presents with a red, non-tender scrotal
mass present at birth. Testicular gangrene is present and the testis subsequently
atrophies. Surgical treatment is usually of no avail in salvaging the infarcted
testis.

In young males, torsion may occur in a normally placed testis and is a recognized complication in testicular maldescent. Torsion usually occurs at adolescence but may present in young males between the ages of 12 and 18 years. The testis which is liable to torsion lies horizontally in the scrotal sac, has a long mesorchium and a long portion of the cord within the vaginal sac (*Fig.* 9.5).

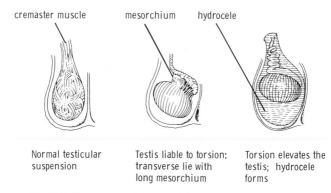

cremaster muscle   mesorchium   hydrocele

| Normal testicular suspension | Testis liable to torsion; transverse lie with long mesorchium | Torsion elevates the testis; hydrocele forms |

Fig. 9.5 Transverse-lying mobile testis liable to torsion.

Clinical Features

Sudden onset of severe acute pain and swelling of the testis with vomiting. There may be a history of previous bouts of testicular pain. On examination, the affected testis is extremely tender and elevated due to shortening of the cord. Palpation of the other side may reveal a horizontal lie and thickening of the cord.

Torsion of the Appendages of the Testis

These are vestigial structures within the scrotum (*Fig.* 9.6):

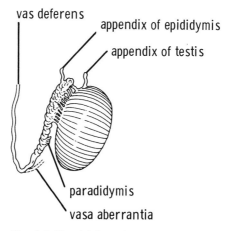

vas deferens

appendix of epididymis

appendix of testis

paradidymis

vasa aberrantia

Fig. 9.6 Vestigial testicular appendages.

1.   Appendix of testis (hydatid of Morgagni).
2.   Appendix of epididymis.
3.   Paradidymis (organ of Giraldes).
4.   Vasa aberrantia (organ of Häller).
     The signs and symptoms of torsion of these vestigial structures are indistinguishable from those of testicular torsion.
Idiopathic Scrotal Oedema
Allergic reaction of the scrotal skin with redness and swelling both sides and of the thigh with pyrexia. The testicles, though impalpable, are normal.

Diagnosis of Torsion
Diagnosis is made on clinical grounds. A Döppler scan may show absent blood flow in the infarcted testis.

Treatment
When a diagnosis of torsion is made, or even suspected, immediate exploration, detorsion and fixation are indicated within 8 hr of the event. After 8 hr the infarcted testis will not recover function and atrophy will result. Attempts at manual detorsion are possible, but must not delay operative treatment. When the testis has been infarcted for over 12 hr an orchidectomy is indicated. Fixation of the contra-lateral testis is indicated at time of the primary operation or 2–3 months later.

●   C. Inflammation of the Epididymis and Testis
1.   Acute epididymo-orchitis—
          Specific—gonorrhea.
          Non-specific—*E. coli, Staphylococcus, Streptococcus.*
2.   Chronic epididymitis—
          Specific—tuberculosis.
          Non-specific—*E. coli, Staphylococcus, Streptococcus.*

Pathology
     The epididymis is involved by retrograde spread from the prostate and seminal vesicles (50 per cent) or by blood-borne infection (50 per cent). The inflamed epididymis secondarily infects the testis: primary orchitis is rare except in association with pancreatitis or mumps (mumps orchitis—18 per cent show testicular involvement).

Predisposing Factors
1.   Operations on the prostate and urethra.
2.   Post-instrumental and post-catheterization.
3.   Mumps, gonorrhoea, typhoid and paratyphoid.
4.   Idiopathic (70 per cent).

Acute Epididymo-orchitis
1.   Resolution—85 per cent resolve on antibiotics.
2.   Secondary hydrocele.
3.   Involvement of scrotal skin.
4.   Discharging scrotal sinuses.
5.   Sloughing of testis—hernia testis.
6.   Testicular atrophy in 20 per cent.
7.   Sterility in bilateral cases.

Clinical Features
Acute onset of pain in testis, fever and rigors. The inflamed organ becomes swollen, red and acutely tender, with rapid development of a hydrocele. In untreated cases scrotal sinuses, discharging pus, may occur after 1 week of acute inflammation.

Differential Diagnosis
In patients under 20 years of age an acute epididymo-orchitis must be distinguished from a torsion of the testis.

Diagnosis
1.   Blood count—leucocytosis.
2.   Blood culture—may be positive for organisms.
3.   Urinalysis—pus cells and organisms.
4.   Döppler scan—normal or increased blood flow in testis.

Treatment
1.   Conservative in 95 per cent of patients—bed rest, scrotal elevation and antibiotic treatment.
2.   Surgery in 5 per cent:
           Incision of a scrotal abscess.
           Excision of scrotal sinuses.
           Orchidectomy in advanced cases.

Chronic Epididymitis
1.   Commonest cause tuberculosis. Others: non-specific infection and filariasis.
2.   Retrograde spread from prostate and seminal vesicles.
3.   Cold abscess of scrotum—multiple scrotal sinuses.
4.   Beading of the vas.
5.   Craggy epididymis.
6.   Hard, irregular seminal vesicle on rectal examination.
Note: All these chronic lesions of tuberculosis are painless.

Treatment
1.   Antituberculous drugs—cure most of the genital lesions of tuberculosis.
2.   Tuberculous sinuses—excision combined with epididymectomy.
3.   Orchidectomy—rarely in intractable cases.

- ### D. Hydrocele: Epididymal Cysts: Spermatocele: Varicocele

Scrotal Swellings

A swelling of the scrotum may be due to:
1. Enlargement of the testis and epididymis—cysts or tumour.
2. Fluid in the vaginal sac around the testis—hydrocele.
3. Descent of abdominal contents through the inguinal canal into the scrotum—hernia.

Clinical differentiation between these three conditions rests on:
1. Ability to get above swelling and palpate a normal cord.
2. Cough impulse in the groin or reduction of a scrotal mass with gurgling.
3. Gentle palpation of the testis and epididymis for discrete lesions or generalized non-tender enlargement of testis.
4. Transillumination of the scrotal mass in a darkened room.

Development of the Vaginal Sac, Hernia and Hydrocele

During the last month of intrauterine life a sac of peritoneum, the processus vaginalis, accompanies the descending testis into the scrotum (*Fig.* 9.1). Complete obliteration of the upper two-thirds of the processus occurs before birth but the distal third remains as an investing sac around the testis and epididymis within the scrotum (tunica vaginalis).
1. Persistence of proximal third of processus—congenital hernia.
2. Persistence of middle third of processus:
    Male—encysted hydrocele of cord.
    Female—hydrocele of canal of Nuck (*Fig.* 9.7).
3. Persistence of whole of processus:
    Congenital hydrocele.
    Inguinoscrotal hernia (*Fig.* 9.8).

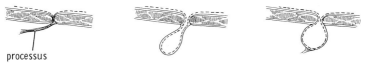

processus

Obliterated processus vaginalis   Congenital hernial sac   Hydrocele of canal of Nuck

Fig. 9.7 Results of defective obliteration of processus vaginalis in female.

Hydrocele

A hydrocele may be congenital or acquired.

Congenital Hydrocele

A congenital hydrocele results from persistence of the processus which allows peritoneal fluid to escaspe into the scrotum. The infant will have an enlarged scrotal sac, often bilateral, and the fluid content is easily demonstrated by transillumination. Most congenital hydroceles resolve by the age of 3 years. Persistence of the hydrocele after 3 years of age is an indication for operative

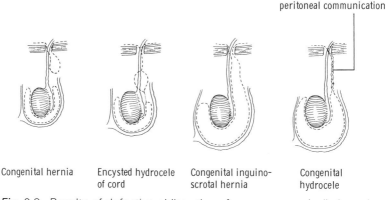

peritoneal communication

Congenital hernia   Encysted hydrocele   Congenital inguino-   Congenital
                    of cord   scrotal hernia   hydrocele

Fig. 9.8. Results of defective obliteration of processus vaginalis in male.

treatment. The operation is a simple division and ligation of the patent processus vaginalis via a groin incision. The vaginal portion of the sac need not be excised. A congenital encysted hydrocele of the cord transilluminates and is treated by simple excision.

Acquired Adult Hydrocele
1.   Primary (idiopathic)—90 per cent.
2.   Secondary—infection, trauma, torsion, tumour—10 per cent.
                The cause of a primary idiopathic hydrocele is lymphatic obstruction
                        to fluid absorption from the scrotal sac.
                Bleeding into the sac—haematocele.
                Secondary infection of the hydrocele fluid—calcification.
                Many idiopathic hydroceles reach an enormous size and contain
                        amber-coloured fluid rich in cholesterol.
                Clinically, the swelling is firm to hard, painless, transilluminates and
                        it is possible to get above the swelling.

Treatment
1.   Elderly and chronic sick patients—repeated needle aspiration.
2.   Fit patients—operation—hydrocelectomy (*Fig.* 9.9).
        Secondary hydroceles are associated with trauma to, or pathology of, the

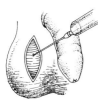

Scrotal incision. Aspiration   Delivery and excision of anterior   Suturing edge of excised sac
of fluid   wall of sac   (haemostatic)

Fig. 9.9 Hydrocelectomy.

contained testis and cord. Hydrocele formation is common with epididymo-orchitis and resolution occurs on antibiotic therapy. Blood in a hydrocele (haematocele) is found in trauma, torsion and some testicular tumours. Treatment of this type of hydrocele is directed towards the primary lesion producing blood in the vaginal fluid.

Epididymal Cysts and Spermatoceles

Single, multiple or multilocular cysts may occur in relation to the epididymis, usually its head. The fluid in the cysts may be clear (epididymal cyst) or turbid and milky (spermatocele), containing spermatozoa. Both epididymal cysts and spermatoceles transilluminate light and may attain sizeable proportions. Testicular palpation differentiates between a spermatocele and a hydrocele. In the former the testis is below and separate from the scrotal mass, whilst in the latter it is incorporated in the posterior wall of the hydrocele sac and its position can only be ascertained by elicitation of testicular sensation (*Fig.* 9.10).

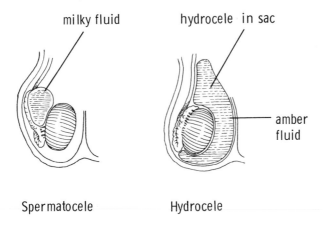

Fig. 9.10 Clinical differentiation between a hydrocele and spermatocele.

Treatment

A small epididymal cyst or spermatocele will not require treatment. Larger cysts may be painful and unsightly and excision is advised in most patients (*Fig.* 9.11).

Varicocele

A varicocele is a varicose condition of the veins of the pampiniform plexus surrounding the cord and testis:
1. Found in 8 per cent of normal males.
2. Left-sided in 90 per cent.
3. Acute onset of left-sided varicocele occurs in 0·004 per cent of patients with a carcinoma of the left kidney.
4. Associated with oligospermia in a few subfertile males.

Clinical Features

1. Dragging pain and aching in the affected testis.
2. Palpation—bag of worms.

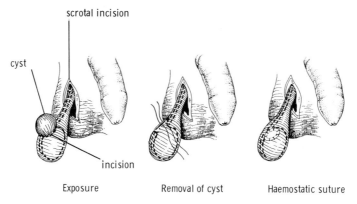

scrotal incision

cyst

incision

Exposure   Removal of cyst   Haemostatic suture

Fig. 9.11 Excision of a spermatocele or a large epididymal cyst.

3.   Cough impulse may be elicited.
4.   Elevation of the scrotum empties the veins.
5.   Thermography may reveal an elevation in skin temperature over the testis on the affected side.

Treatment
1.   In patients with severe aching and discomfort—varicocelectomy.
2.   For subfertility group—operative excision.

●   **E. Tumours of the Testis**
Benign tumours of the testis are extremely rare. Historically, the syphylitic gumma was a differential diagnosis—hardly ever seen in modern practice.

Malignant Testicular Tumours

Aetiology
1.   History of trauma in some patients—probably not significant.
2.   Maldescended testis has a 40 times greater chance of developing a malignant tumour as compared with a normally descended testis.

Incidence
1.   3 per 100 000 white males in Europe and N. America.
2.   Rare in Negroes, including N. American Negroes.
3.   Steady unexplained increase in incidence over past 20 years.
4.   Rare before puberty
        Teratoma—peak incidence 20–30 years.
        Seminoma—peak incidence 30–40 years.
        Lymphoma—elderly males.

Pathology
Frequency of each type of primary tumour:
1.   Seminoma   —40 per cent.
2.   Teratoma   —34 per cent.
3.   Combined seminoma and teratoma—14 per cent.
4.   Lymphoma   — 7 per cent.
5.   Tumour rarities   — 5 per cent.
     Secondary tumours of the testis are extremely rare. Testicular tumour deposits may occur in leukaemia.
     The germ cell gives rise to all malignant tumours of the testis.
1.   Germ cell—seminoma.
2.   Germ cell—embryonal carcinoma:
          Interstitial cell
          Sertoli cell
          Yolk sac (orchidoblastoma).
          Endo-, meso- and ectoderm—teratoma.

Staging of Testicular Tumours
Histological staging depends on degree of differentiation of the tumour cells.
     A pure seminoma is always well differentiated (universal stage).
     Teratoma staging:
1.   TD—well-differentiated cells.
2.   MTI—differentiation and early malignant change.
3.   MTU—no differentiation.
4.   MTT—poor differentiation and elements of MTI amd MTU.

Clinical Staging
Clinical staging relies on clinical examination, with radiological evidence of lymph node involvement and distant metastases.
1.   Stage   I—tumour in testis.
2.   Stage   II—tumour in testis and para-aortic nodes.
3.   Stage III—tumour in testis, para-aortic, mediastinal and supraclavicular nodes.
4.   Stage IV—stage III with liver or bony metastases.

Spread of Tumour
Lymphatic to para-aortic nodes and external iliac nodes. Later spread to mediastinal and supraclavicular nodes (*Fig.* 9.12). Blood-stream metastases to lungs and liver occur late, with exception of MTT teratoma which may produce early multiple distant metastases (hurricane dissemination).
     Tumour involvement of scrotal skin is a very late method of spread.

Clinical Features
Presenting symptoms include:
1.   Painless swelling of the testis—80 per cent.
2.   Sensation of weight in the testis and aching—10 per cent.
3.   No symptoms—chance discovery—5 per cent.
4.   Distant metastases in lymph node, lung or liver—15 per cent.

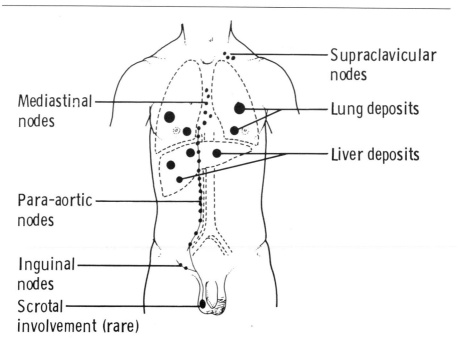

Mediastinal nodes

Supraclavicular nodes

Lung deposits

Liver deposits

Para-aortic nodes

Inguinal nodes

Scrotal involvement (rare)

Fig. 9.12 Dissemination of a malignant testicular tumour.

Examination
1. Enlarged, hard, painless swelling with diminished or absent testicular sensation.
2. Associated with a lax hydrocele in 12 per cent of patients.
3. Rapidly growing teratoma may show inflammatory changes.
4. Palpate abdomen for para-aortic lymph node enlargement and evidence of liver metastases.
5. Examine neck for supraclavicular node enlargement.
6. Routine examination of the chest for evidence of pulmonary metastases.

Investigations
1. *Preoperative*:

    Chest X-ray—pulmonary metastases (*Fig.* 9.13).
    Blood—tumour markers:
    aFP (alpha-feto protein).
    BHCG (beta-chorionic gonadotrophin).
    aFP:
    Not detectable in seminoma.
    Elevated in teratoma.
    BHCG:
    Present in 5 per cent seminoma.
    Elevated in 90 per cent teratoma.

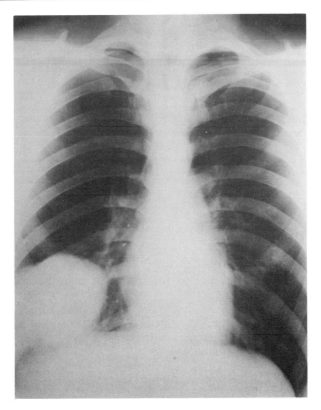

Fig. 9.13 'Cannon-ball' secondary lung deposits in a patient with a testicular tumour.

2.　*Postoperative*:

Investigations for lymph node involvement and distant metastases:

IVU—ureteric displacement by para-aortic nodes.

Lymphography—detection of lymph node metastases (*Fig.* 6.18).

Ultrasound scan—abdominal lymph node masses.

CT scan—abdominal node enlargement.

Repeat blood tumour markers:

Evidence of residual active tumour.

After primary treatment.

Treatment— General Principles

1.　A testicular tumour must be excised by orchidectomy (*Fig.* 9.14).
2.　A testicular tumour must never be biopsied.
3.　Orchidectomy is combined with either radiotherapy or chemotherapy for tumour metastases.
4.　Seminoma is very radiosensitive.

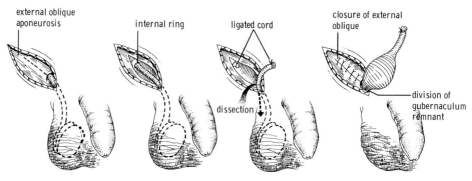

Fig. 9.14 Orchidectomy.

Treatment–Specific

1.   Seminoma:

        Stage   I—radiotherapy to para-aortic nodes in all cases.

        Stage   II—radiotherapy to para-aortic nodes + mediastinal and supraclavicular nodes.

        Stages III and IV—radiotherapy and chemotherapy.

        Stages I and II tumours—95 per cent 5-year survival.

2.   Teratoma:

        Stage   I—chemotherapy.

        Stage   II—chemotherapy + surgical excision of residual lymph nodes.

        Stages III and IV—chemotherapy.

        Stages I and II tumours—80 per cent 5-year survival.

        Stages III and IV tumours—10 per cent 5-year survival.

Note:

    Combination chemotherapy is supervised in special centres.

    Combination drugs used—vinblastine, bleomycin and *cis*-platinum.

●   **F. Male Infertility: Impotence: Sterilization**

Male Infertility

    The urologist is asked on occasions to determine fertility in the male in a childless marriage after the ability of the female partner to conceive has been demonstrated by a gynaecologist.

Significant Clinical History

1.   Venereal disease.
2.   Epididymo-orchitis.
3.   Mumps.
4.   Hernia or scrotal operations.
5.   Disorder of sexual function.

6.   Drugs, alcoholism, smoking.

Examination of Genitalia
1.   Position, size and consistency of testes.
2.   Presence of varicocele (90 per cent left-sided).
3.   Palpation of vasa.
4.   Rectal examination.

Investigations
        Semen analysis (normal values).
            Volume—2–6 ml.
            Sperm population—20 millions/ml:
                60 per cent motile sperm.
                60 per cent morphologically normal.
      Note:
                Presence of pus cells is abnormal.
                Oligospermia—reduced sperm population.
            Azoospermia—absence of spermatozoa.

Specific Tests
1.   Follicular stimulating hormone (FSH) level.
2.   Plasma testosterone level.
3.   Leutinizing hormone (LH) level.
4.   Antisperm antibody:
        Present in seminal fluid or cervical mucus and produces measurable
        blood levels in some infertile patients.
5.   Testicular biopsy:
        Indicator of normal, abnormal or absent spermatogenesis.
6.   Vasography:
        Injection of radio-opaque dye into vas at open operation demon-
        strates patency of vasa.
7.   Scrotal thermography:
        Identification of a varicocele.

Treatment
1.   General:
        Loose undergarments.
        Abstain from alcohol, drugs and smoking.
        Regular intercourse, 3 times a week.
2.   Presence of antisperm antibodies with normal sperm count:
        Low dose steroid.
        AIH (artificial insemination by husband).
3.   Oligospermia:
        Ligation of varicocele, if present.
4.   Azoospermia:
        Elevated FSH and small testes—AID (artificial insemination by
        donor).
        Normal FSH and normal testes—blockage of vasa—epididymo-
        vasostomy.

Impotence

Inability to achieve or maintain an erection, making satisfactory intercourse impossible.

Impotence is organic or psychogenic:

1. Social—drug abuse, alcoholism, advance in years.
2. Organic causes:

    Medical—diabetes, tabes dorsalis, spinal cord lesions.

    Surgical—abdomino-perineal resection: aorto-iliac surgery.

There is no satisfactory treatment for any of these forms of impotence. An artificial penile prosthesis may be used in patients in the younger age groups.

Male Sterilization

Vasectomy in the male has become a popular method of contraception.

Indications

1. Medical:

    In the male:

    Hereditary disease, e.g. Huntington's chorea.

    In the female:

    Medical reasons for not having further pregnancies, e.g. toxaemia, repeated Caesarean sections.

2. Social:

    Between 28 and 45 years.

    Stable marriage.

    Family of two or more children.

    No history of psychogenic or sexual aberration.

    Economic grounds.

Counselling

1. Consent of both partners to operation.
2. Operation regarded as irreversible.
3. Necessity for two azoospermic counts after operation.

Reasons for Failure

1. Technical at primary operation.
2. Recanalization of ligated vasa.

    Most vasectomy operations are performed under local anaesthetic.

Vasectomy Reversal (Vaso-vasostomy)

1. Technically difficult.
2. 50 per cent chance of return of sperm to seminal fluid.
3. 30 per cent chance of fertility.
4. Antisperm antibodies occasionally appear after a successful vasectomy reversal procedure.

10

Urinary drainage: urinary diversion

● **A. Urinary Drainage**

Temporary decompression or drainage of the urinary tract is frequently employed in urological practice. Drainage entails the insertion of a tube or catheter into the kidney and renal pelvis (nephrostomy and pyelostomy), into the ureter (intubated ureterostomy), into the bladder (suprapubic cystostomy and cutaneous vesicostomy) and retrogradely into the bladder via a perineal urethrostomy or urethral catheter (*Fig.* 10.1).

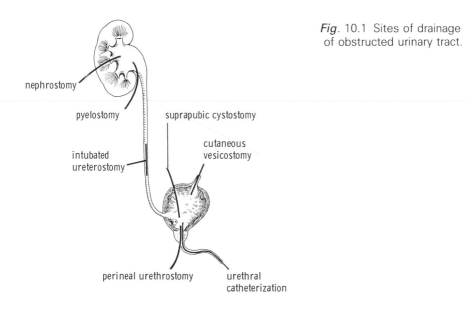

Fig. 10.1 Sites of drainage of obstructed urinary tract.

nephrostomy

pyelostomy

suprapubic cystostomy

intubated ureterostomy

cutaneous vesicostomy

perineal urethrostomy

urethral catheterization

The two complications of a drainage tube in contact with urine are:
1. Infection.
2. Stone formation due to crystallization of urates on the catheter.

These complications were a common feature with the use of rubber catheters, with an added long-term complication of stricture formation due to the chemical urethritis induced by the rubber. Modern catheters are constructed of polyvinyl plastic materials (Silastic) which are only marginally irritant to the urothelium and are less prone to stimulate the deposition of urates on the portion of the catheter in contact with urine. Silastic catheters may be used for long-term decompression and drainage of the urinary tract.

Nephrostomy
    Nephrostomy is a temporary measure to decompress the renal pelvis proximal to a distal obstruction. A pyelostomy and intubated ureterostomy are rarely used in modern practice. The nephrostomy may be constructed at open operation or, more commonly, introduced percutaneously under ultrasound control using a pig-tail catheter. Nephrostomy tubes are removed as soon as the distal obstruction has been surgically relieved. Permanent nephrostomy drainage is rarely indicated and if employed, the Tressider method (*Fig.* 10.2) is advocated.

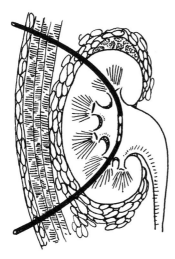

Fig. 10.2. Tressider method of nephrostomy.

Cystostomy
    Cystostomy may be achieved by suprapubic catheterization or urethral catheterization. A perineal urethrostomy is seldom employed in modern urological practice. Urethral catheterization is the commonest method of draining the bladder. Suprapubic needle puncture may be used for obtaining a clean specimen of urine for culture in the obstructed infant bladder. Suprapubic catheterization is a temporary method of drainage in patients with bladder outflow obstruction. In both methods of drainage the catheter must be introduced under full sterile precautions.
    Permanent indwelling bladder drainage is sometimes necessary in elderly, sick or incontinent patients and in these groups a Silastic catheter changed every 8 weeks is employed, or alternatively a cutaneous vesicostomy as described by Lapides (*Fig.* 10.3) is fashioned. In the majority of patients who need permanent catheterization some form of urinary diversion is advised, but in many with

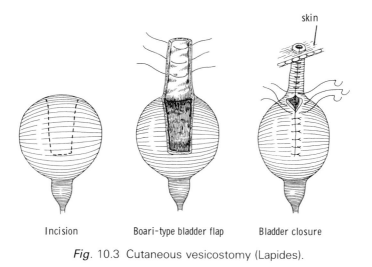

Incision   Boari-type bladder flap   Bladder closure

Fig. 10.3 Cutaneous vesicostomy (Lapides).

acquired neurogenic lesions intermittent self-catheterization or a permanent indwelling catheter is the drainage method of choice.

● B. Urinary Diversion

Methods of Diversion

Diversion of urine from its normal course to the exterior via the urethra may be achieved by:
1. Bringing the ureters to the skin surface.
2. Anastomosing the ureters to an intact intestinal tract.
3. Use of intestinal conduits or reservoir drainage to the skin surface.
   The methods of urinary diversion are tabulated below:
1. Diversion by ureterostomy:
   Bilateral   —two stomata.
   Loop   —one or two stomata.
   Double-barrelled   —one stoma.
   Transuretero-ureterostomy—one stoma.
2. Sphincter-preserving diversion:
   Uretero-sigmoidostomy.
   Rectal bladder (Mauclaire).
   Gersuny operation.
3. Diversion by conduit (non-sphincteric):
   Ileal loop conduit.
   Sigmoid loop conduit.

Ureterostomy
1. Rarely employed—nephrostomy is preferred.

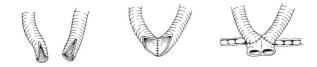

Spatulation of ureters   Side-to-side anastomosis   Twin ureterostomy

Fig. 10.4 Double-barrelled ureterostomy.

2.   Loop ureteostomy used in infants with long tortuous ureters.
3.   Double-barrelled ureterostomy and a single stoma (*Fig.* 10.4) may on occasions be used in infants for permanent drainage in bladder outlet obstruction.
4.   Transuretero-ureterostomy (*Fig.* 10.5) may also be used in similar circumstances with the formation of a single stoma.

I. V. C.   *Fig*. 10.5 Transuretero-ureterostomy.

Aorta

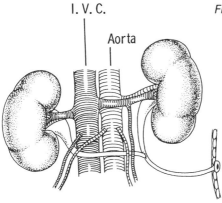

Uretero-sigmoidostomy

A time-honoured method of diversion in which the divided ureters are anastomosed to the sigmoid colon in a reflux-preventing manner, the urine subsequently passing to the exterior mixed with the faecal stream. The continent rectum and distal sigmoid colon act as a common reservoir for urine and faeces (*Fig.* 10.6). Modifications of this operation are described by Mauclaire, in which the ureters are anastomosed to an isolated rectal reservoir and a colostomy is fashioned (*Fig.* 10.7) and Gersuny, in which the colostomy is brought through the anal sphincter muscles in common with the urinary conduit from the isolated rectal reservoir (*Fig.* 10.8).

Ileal and Sigmoid Loop Conduits

The ileal loop conduit was introduced by Bricker in 1955 for urinary diversion. An isolated vascularized loop of terminal ileum is brought to the skin of the abdominal wall to form a stoma and the divided ureters are anastamosed to this loop, either separately or after approximation of the ends of the ureters to form a

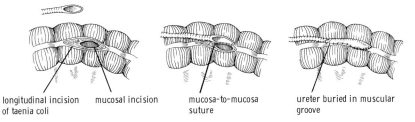

longitudinal incision   mucosal incision   mucosa-to-mucosa   ureter buried in muscular
of taenia coli   suture   groove

Fig. 10.6 Ureterosigmoidostomy.

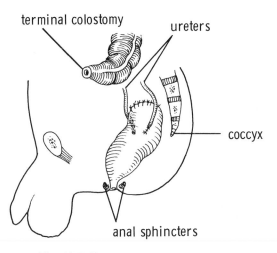

Fig. 10.7 Rectal bladder (Mauclaire).

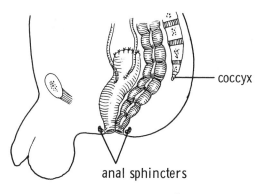

Fig. 10.8 Gersuny operation.

common tube (*Fig* 10.9). In a similar fashion, the mid-part of the sigmoid colon may be used as the conduit (Mogg). An important feature of both these operations for urinary diversion is the siting and fashioning of the cutaneous stoma. Most of the complications of urinary diversion arise from problems with the cutaneous stoma.

Indications for Urinary Diversion
1.   Alternative pathway for urinary drainage in a patient with intractable incontinence due to a spina bifida or acquired neurogenic bladder lesions.
2.   Exernal conduit for urine following surgical ablation of the lower urinary tract or following irradiation, fibrosis of the pelvic organs or irresectable tumours of the bladder, rectum and uterus.
3.   Method of drainage following irreparable injury, obstruction or disease of the lower urinary tract.

Complications of Urinary Diversion after Uretero-sigmoidostomy
1.   Ascending infection:
              Chronic pyelonephritis and renal failure (40 per cent).
2.   Electrolytic imbalance:
              Reabsorption of urinary constituents from the bowel, producing hyperchloraemic acidosis (50 per cent).

Complications after Ileal or Sigmoid Conduits
1.   Hyperchloraemic acidosis (15 per cent).
2.   Stomal problems (40 per cent).

Management of Complications

Hyperchloraemic acidosis:
         Acute.
         Chronic.
Acute Hyperchloraemic Acidosis
Often presents with mental confusion and disorientation or coma: to be differentiated from diabetic coma or barbiturate poisoning.
         Treatment includes adequate drainage of the urinary reservoir, intravenous infusion of molar lactate solution (an alkaline agent) and antibiotic therapy.
Chronic Hyperchloraemic Acidosis
May manifest itself within months or years of the diversionary operation and prone to occur in patients with renal damage prior to operation and in those with urinary retention in the conduit.
         Symptoms—thirst, anorexia, nausea, vomiting, weight loss, muscular weakness, mental confusion, coma and death, if untreated. Skeletal changes (renal osteodystrophy) with bone pain and pathological fractures may supervene in long-standing chronic hyperchloraemic acidosis.
         Treatment—as for the acute condition. Surgical revision of the conduit may be necessary. A uretero-sigmoidostomy procedure should be converted into an ileal loop conduit.

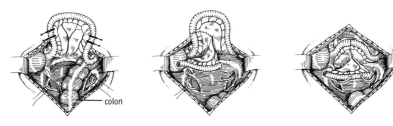

Isolation of ileal loop.	Closure of left end of loop.	Implantation of the ureters
Mobilization of ureters.	Left ureter brought through	into the isolated ileal loop
	transverse mesocolon	

Fig. 10.9 Ileal-loop conduit (Bricker).

Stomal Problems

Bleeding, retraction, prolapse, intussusception, torsion and incrustation with squamous type epithelium.

Treatment—reconstruction procedures for the stoma and resiting of the stoma. Rarely—creation of a new conduit.

Note:

Ileal or sigmoid loop patients with hyperchloraemic acidosis may have a long loop and the condition is often reversed by resection and shortening of the conduit.

Selection of Diversionary Procedure

1. In children:

    Exstrophy of bladder—ileal loop conduit.
    Neurogenic bladder—ileal loop conduit.
    Dilated tortuous ureters—transuretero-ureterostomy.

2. In adults:

    Non-malignant conditions—ileal loop conduit.
    Vesico-vaginal fistulae (malignant)—ileal loop conduit.
    Neurogenic incontinence—ileal loop conduit.
    Intractable urethral strictures—ileal or sigmoid loop conduit.
    Pelvic malignancy—radical treatment—ileal loop conduit.
    Pelvic malignancy—palliative:
        Good anal sphincter—uretero-sigmoidostomy
        Poor sphincter—ileal conduit.

Prognosis of Diversionary Operations

1. Diversionary ileal conduit:

    Operative mortality—4 per cent.
    Operative morbidity:
        Hyperchloraemic acidosis—15 per cent.
        Stomal problems—40 per cent.

2. Uretero-sigmoidostomy:

    Operative mortality—4 per cent.
    Operative morbidity:
        Pyelonephritis—40 per cent.
        Hyperchloraemic acidosis—50 per cent.

In both types of operation the prognosis will depend largely on the functional state of the kidneys prior to operation and on the basic pathology for which the operation has been advised. In terms of morbidity the ileal loop or sigmoid loop conduit is a much safer procedure than a uretero-sigmoidostomy. The uretero-sigmoidostomy procedure should be reserved for palliation of advanced malignant conditions of the pelvic organs in frail and elderly patients with satisfactory anal continence.

Management of renal failure

● **A. Acute and Chronic Renal Failure**
Failure of the kidneys to excrete metabolic waste products from the circulation leads to a clinical state of uraemia. The primary pathological processes producing failure may be intrinsic (intra-renal) or extrinsic (extra-renal) and in some patients failure results from a combination of both these factors. From the clinical standpoint, renal failure may present acutely or may be a culmination of long-standing and gradual deterioration of renal function (chronic renal failure: CRF: end-stage renal disease).

Acute Renal Failure (ARF)
In acute failure, excretory function of the kidneys is rapidly compromised with gross disruption of blood chemistry, oliguria and occasionally anuria.
Aetiological classification:
Pre-renal.
Renal.
Post-renal.

Pre-renal Failure
Any condition which limits renal circulation and glomerular perfusion may cause acute deterioration of renal function. Renal circulation is curtailed in the state of shock due to vasoconstriction of the renal arteries (renal shut-down mechanism).
Causes of pre-renal uraemia include:
1. Trauma, especially crush injuries.
2. Burns.
3. Major haemorrhage or fluid loss.
4. Obstetric complications.
5. Gram-negative septicaemia.
6. Acute pancreatitis.
7. Liver disease and jaundice.
8. Hypercalcaemia.

Renal Causes
1. Acute tubular necrosis:
Obstetric catastrophes, eclampsia, abortion.
Major surgery:
Resection of aortic aneurysm.

        Cardiac surgery.

        Acute pancreatitis.

        Drugs and poisons—nephrotoxic agents—mercury, gold, chlorates.

        Advanced liver disease—hepato-renal failure.

        Leukaemia and myeloma.

2.   Primary glomerulo-nephritis:

        Poly-arteritis nodosa.

        Systemic lupus erythematosus.

3.   Renal vascular disease:

        Malignant hypertension.

        Eclampsia and post-partum haemorrhage.

        Thrombocytopenic purpura.

        Septicaemia.

4.   Acute interstitial nephritis:

        Drug hypersensitivity—

                Penicillin analogues.

                Sulphonamides.

                Phenylbutazone.

                Phenindione.

Post-renal causes

Obstruction is an uncommon cause for acute failure, although ARF occasionally occurs in calculus obstruction or retroperitoneal fibrosis.

    Provided uraemia due to drug therapy, shock or obstructive uropathy can be excluded, the commonest cause for ARF is tubular necrosis. ARF due to tubular necrosis is reversible in most instances, but permanent and more serious renal cortical necrosis may supervene in 2 per cent of patients.

Clinical Features

The early symptoms of ARF are unremarkable and often overshadowed by the primary pathology causing the renal failure. The earliest sign of impending failure is oliguria, the patient excreting less than 400 ml of urine in 24 hr. Later symptoms are those of uraemia:

1.   Gastro-intestinal—anorexia, nausea, vomiting, diarrhoea.
2.   Muscular—cramps, flapping tremor of muscles.
3.   Coagulation deficiencies—bruising, gastro-intestinal bleeding, pericarditis.
4.   Cerebral—lethargy, diminished consciousness, coma.
5.   Vascular—hypotension and fainting on standing.
6.   Pulmonary—oedema.
7.   Anaemia—occurs early: secondary to bone marrow depression.

Note:

    Patients in ARF are very prone to systemic infection, which is the ultimate cause of death in most patients.

Diagnosis

Clinical suspicion in a patient after major injury or surgery with oliguria.

1.   Urinalysis:

        Urine of low specific gravity containing protein and red cells.

2.   Blood chemistry:
     Rising blood urea and plasma creatinine: rise in blood urea of 5 mmol/l per day indicates progressive failure.
     Hyperkalaemia:
          Elevation of plasma potassium over 6 mmol/l may cause myocardial irritability and ventricular fibrillation.
     Hypocalcaemia and phosphate retention.
     Hyponatraemia:
          Depression of sodium level—often compensated by over-transfusion with i.v. fluids.

Management of ARF
Management is medical and in most instances the condition is reversible.
1.   Accurate maintenance of fluid intake and output—fluid balance charts.
2.   Protein-free diet—carbohydrate diet with vitamin supplements.
3.   Correction of anaemia—small transfusions of packed fresh blood.
4.   Prompt systemic antibiotic therapy, if infection is present.
5.   Urgent treatment of hyperkalaemia (with ECG evidence of cardiac irregularities)—glucose and insulin infusion: i.v. calcium.
6.   Early dialysis before blood urea reaches 30 mmol/l and repeated at intervals to keep the blood urea below this level.
7.   Avoid nephrotoxic drugs—tetracycline; combination of gentamycin and cephaloridine.
8.   Parenteral feeding in severely ill patients.
     ARF lasts for 3 days to 3–4 weeks. After complete recovery 10–20 per cent of the nephrons will be lost but there is no permanent deterioration in renal function. Mortality rate of ARF is increased in patients over 60 years of age, irrespective of aetiology of the failure:

Mortality in surgical cases:

Pregnancy and abortion	10–20 per cent.
Major surgery and trauma	50–60 per cent.
Major burns	70 per cent.
Mortality in all medical cases — all causes	30–40 per cent.

     The major factors in mortality are sepsis and gastro-intestinal haemorrhage. Prognosis for ARF has been vastly improved by the use of early and repeated dialysis.

Chronic Renal Failure (CRF)
     Chronic renal failure is the result of progressive disease of, or obstruction to, both kidneys which interferes with their capacity to maintain normal electrolytic equilibrium of the body fluids.

Incidence and Aetiology
Annual death rate in Great Britain per annum from renal disease is over 7000, and 35–40 new patients in CRF per million population will be candidates for renal dialysis and renal transplantation.

The conditions which produce CRF are either medical or surgical:
CRF medical:
>Chronic pyelonephritis.
>Chronic glomerulonephritis.
>Hypertensive renal disease.
>Polycystic kidneys.
>Renal tuberculosis.
>Metabolic diseases
>>Diabetes, gout, amyloid, hypercalcaemia, cystinosis.
>Lupus erythematosus.

CRF surgical:
>Congenital renal dysplasia.
>Chronic obstructive uropathy.
>Renal calculus disease.
>Retroperitoneal fibrosis.

Effects of CRF
These include:
>Primary—destruction and malfunction of glomeruli and tubules.
>Secondary—anaemia, hypertension, oesteodystrophy.

Primary Renal Effects
Inefficiency of the glomeruli leads to diminution in the rate of glomerular filtration and retention of urea. Tubular dysfunction is reflected in disturbances in water and sodium output, potassium excretion and hydrogen ion concentration.
1. The kidneys excrete dilute urine.
2. Salt and water retention—oedema and cardiac failure.
3. Hyponatraemia—sodium leak.
4. Hyperkalaemia—potassium retention.
5. Failure to reabsorb bicarbonate—metabolic acidosis.
6. Hypocalcaemia—defective metabolism of vitamin D.

Secondary Renal Effects
1. Hypochromic anaemia is a constant factor in CRF.
2. Anaemia
>Lack of erythropoietic hormone.
>Haemolysis and bleeding tendency.
3. Hypertension—renal ischaemia—release of renin.
4. Osteodystrophy:
>Persistent hypocalcaemia stimulates absorption of calcium salts from bones—softening and cyst formation (osteomalacia).

Symptoms and Signs of CRF
Progressive CRF is insidious in appearance and the effects on the patient are those of uraemia combined with systemic manifestations (*Table* 11.1).

Diagnosis of CRF
In the majority of patients a clinical diagnosis of CRF is possible:
1. Urinalysis—proteinuria, casts and occasional red cells.
2. Blood—hypochromic anaemia.
3. Blood urea—grossly elevated > 20 mmol/l.

Table 11.1. Symptoms and signs of CRF

System	Symptoms	Signs
Cardiovascular	Palpitations, dyspnoea, chest pains, epistaxis, headaches	Hypertension, cardiomegaly, pericarditis, heart failure
Ocular	Blurring of vision	Papilloedema
Respiratory	Dyspnoea, haemoptysis, pleurisy	Pleural effusion, congestion, sighing respirations
Gastro-intestinal	Anorexia, nausea, vomiting, hiccups, diarrhoea	Halitosis, ascites, hepatosplenomegaly
Haematological	Tiredness, lethargy, bleeding tendency	Anaemia, bruising
Neurological	Drowsiness, tremors, convulsions, leg cramps	Hyperactive reflexes, coma
Muscular	Joint pains, muscle wasting	Loss of ankle jerk, wasting
Skin	Pruritis, dryness	Pallor, yellow pigmentation
Endocrine	Loss of libido, amenorrhoea, infertility	Oligospermia, gynaecomastia, metropathia

The early symptoms of CRF are lethargy, tiredness, tremors, lack of libido, deterioration of intellectual powers, pallor and dryness of skin, anorexia, halitosis and weight loss. The patient will be anaemic, will have a 'uraemic' odour of the breath and may be hypertensive.

4. Serum creatinine—grossly elevated > 90 μmol/l.
5. IVU—often unrewarding due to poor excretion of dye.
6. Ultrasonography—enlargement of kidneys (obstruction or polycystic disease): small contracted kidneys.
7. DTPA scan—diminished excretion but no stasis or obstruction in contracted kidneys.
8. CT scan—demonstrates size of kidneys.
9. Renal biopsy—only necessary if diagnosis cannot be established.
10. Creatinine clearance test:
    In early CRF clearance is under 10 ml per min.
    In late CRF clearance is below 5 ml per min, and signs and symptoms of CRF will be present.

Management of CRF
Aim of treatment of CRF is to minimize the effects of uraemia and where possible to eliminate the secondary effects on the system. Glomerular filtration rate (GFR) will determine the management policy for patients with established progressive CRF. The creatinine clearance test is a reasonably accurate method of assessing GFR (p. 6).

Treatment Policy
1. GFR > 15 ml per min—asymptomatic patient—no treatment.
2. GFR between 15 and 10 ml per min—early symptoms—dietary treatment.
3. GFR < 10 ml per min—with or without gross symptoms—dialysis and renal transplantation.

Dietary and Medical Treatment

The basis of this form of treatment is a low protein, high carbohydrate intake, with restriction of potassium, addition of vitamins and careful control of fluid intake to balance accurately fluid output each day. Hypertension and congestive cardiac failure will require medical therapy. Secondary anaemia is well tolerated by the patient in CRF and transfusions of fresh blood are reserved for those patients with proven blood loss.

Indications for Dialysis

Patients in CRF:
1. GFR less than 10 ml per min.
2. Plasma creatinine > 90 μmol/l.
3. Clinical signs of peripheral neuropathy, pericarditis or encephalopathy.

Patients accepted for long-term dialysis will be entered on the renal transplantation programme. In Great Britain it is estimated that 40 new CRF patients per million of population present each year with end-stage renal disease, with the implication that 2000 new patients each year need dialysis and renal transplantation. The limiting factors in treating all these patients are lack of space on dialysis units and shortage of kidney donors.

●   **B. Dialysis**

Dialysis refers to the process of extraction of excess waste products from the body fluids. The patient's own peritoneum may be used as a dialysing membrane (peritoneal dialysis) or the blood may be diverted outside the body and redirected through an artificial kidney which extracts the waste products (haemodialysis). Peritoneal dialysis and haemodialysis are two methods employed in the management of patients in CRF. Peritoneal dialysis is sometimes referred to as 'intracorporeal dialysis', whilst the method employing an artificial kidney is called 'extracorporeal dialysis'.

Peritoneal Dialysis

Peritoneal dialysis has been therapeutically available since 1955 and is used in emergency management of acute reversible renal failure and in those patients in CRF awaiting admission to a dialysis unit for haemodialysis. Under full sterile precautions and local anaesthesia, a catheter is introduced into the pelvis and warm dialysing fluid is injected rapidly into the abdominal cavity and withdrawn after 15 min. Dialysis is repeated, the aim being to wash out the peritoneum with 2 litres of fluid every hour for up to 72 hr. The method is very effective and inexpensive (cost £50 per 24 hr dialysis), but the main disadvantage is a significant incidence of sepsis and peritonitis. For this reason treatment must be discontinued after three or four days.

Haemodialysis

Haemodialysis may be employed as a short-term or a long-term therapeutic measure. Short-term dialysis is used for ARF, particularly the

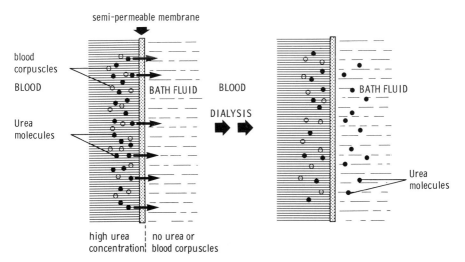

Fig. 11.1 Haemodynamic principles utilized in haemodialysis.

hypercatabolic variety, in the treatment of barbiturate, salicylate or thiocyanate poisoning and in the treatment of severe diabetic ketosis with oliguria. Long-term haemodialysis is employed therapeutically in the management of CRF and as a preliminary and complementary method of management for those patients destined for renal transplantation.

Basic Principles of Haemodialysis
The patient's circulation is connected to an extracorporeal machine in which blood circulates on one side of a semi-permeable membrane and a solution of water and electrolytes on the other side of the same membrane. The membrane is permeable to diffusible substances but impermeable to larger molecules in the circulating plasma. Various diffusible substances in the plasma will perfuse through the dialysing membrane if the concentration of these substances on each side of the membrane is unequal (*Fig.* 11.1). In the extracorporeal machine (artificial kidney) blood is exposed to a vast area of membrane for diffusion. This principle is achieved by coiling the membranes around a rotating drum (Kölff dialyser) or pumping blood into stationary spirals by hydrostatic arterial pressure (Kiil dialyser). The patient is connected to a dialysing machine by cannulating an artery or vein and shunting blood from the artery through the dialyser and back into the vein. The blood entering the dialyser is heparinized to avoid clotting during passage between the membranes in the dialyser. Heparin in the returning blood is neutralized by a protamine infusion. To avoid repeated cannalization of an artery and vein an artificial arteriovenous shunt has been devised (Scribner) in which the artery and vein are permanently joined by a Teflon tube (*Fig.* 11.2). In long-term dialysis the Scribner shunt may become defunct after 6–9 months' usage, or infection may occur at the site of cannalization of the vessels, and the shunt has to be refashioned at another site. If the establishment of numerous Scribner shunts is anticipated, an arteriovenous forearm fistula may be surgically created (*Fig.* 11.2). This leads to distension and arterialization of the

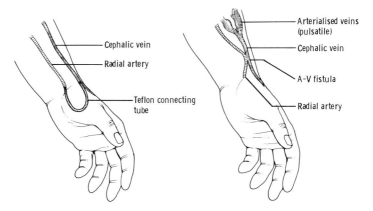

Fig. 11.2 Scribner shunt and arterio-venous forearm fistula.

surrounding veins which may then be utilized for creation of further arteriovenous shunts.

Note:

> For short-term haemodialysis, a Scribner shunt or surgical arterio-venous fistula is not fashioned.

Long-term Haemodialysis

Long-term haemodialysis is undertaken in a dialysis centre or in the patient's home (home dialysis). Treatment is started in hospital where an arteriovenous forearm shunt is created. Suitability of the patient, his/her relatives and his/her house are assessed for the possibility of continuing dialysis in the home. Haemodialysis, both in hospital and in the home, is expensive (a home dialysing unit costs £4000 and its maintenance costs £2500 per annum). In most instances, once a patient has been accepted on a dialysis programme, he or she will be regarded as a potential candidate for renal transplantation.

Complications of Haemodialysis

1. Anaemia:

    > A persistent feature in dialysis patients—treated by oral iron therapy or small volume blood transfusions.

2. Hypertension:

    > Present in 75 per cent of dialysis patients—often improved by dialysis: anti-hypertensive drugs in some instances.

3. Osteodystrophy:

    > 6 per cent—low plasma calcium and elevated plasma phosphate—treated by regulation of calcium and phosphate intake.

4. Hepatitis:

    > In patients and hospital staff in dialysis units: 10 per cent of patients have positive serology for Australia antigen. Outbreaks of hepatitis in dialysis units may lead to closure of the units for lengthy periods.

5. Social problem:
   Patient and family may suffer from psychological trauma of continued home dialysis.
6. Sexual function:
   Depressed in CRF—corrected by dialysis and transplantation.
   Males—impotence.
   Females—lack of libido.
7. Drug therapy:
   Digitalis and amino glycosides avoided.
   Tetracyclines and nephro-toxic drugs not prescribed.

• C. Renal Transplantation

All patients in CRF on a dialysis programme are potential candidates for renal transplantation. The limiting factors in any transplantation unit are lack of haemodialysis facilities for all patients in CRF and the availability of suitable cadaveric kidneys for transplantation.

Development of Renal Transplantation

Transplantation of a cadaveric kidney in a patient with polycystic disease was undertaken by Lawler in 1950 with an unsuccessful outcome. In 1956, Merrill successfully transplanted a kidney in a consanguineous twin. Transplantation of a kidney from a live, related donor to the recipient has been undertaken since this time but, by and large, is not nowadays acceptable on ethical grounds. The main problem in renal transplantation is rejection of the donor kidney by the host but the incidence of rejection was minimized by the introduction of azathioprine as an immunosuppressive agent in 1960. Since the late 1960's, cadaveric kidneys have been used almost exclusively in the management of CRF by renal transplantation.

Demand for Renal Transplantation

In Great Britain it has been estimated that 40 new patients per million population present each year in CRF for dialysis and are potential candidates for renal transplantation. This number, together with those patients who need a second or third transplant for irretrievable host rejection, indicates that about 3000 renal transplants a year are necessary to keep up with demand. Currently, in the UK 1800–2000 transplantation operations are undertaken annually— a short-fall of 1000–1200 patients. The number of transplant operations that can be undertaken is limited by space on a dialysis programme and the availability of suitable donor cadaveric kidneys.

Selection of Patients for Renal Transplantation

Age is no longer a barrier to a transplant operation: patients are accepted between the ages of 5 and 65 years.
Contraindications to transplantation:
1. Chronic sepsis such as bronchiectasis or active tuberculosis.
2. Severe myocardial disease.
3. Advanced neoplastic disease.

4.   Positive Australia antigen patients.

Preparation of Recipient for Transplantation
1.   Elimination of sepsis:
          Treatment of dental caries.
          Treatment of sinus infections.
          Sterilization of urinary tract.
          Surgical removal of infected and functionless kidney.
          Surgical treatment of bladder outlet obstruction.
2.   ABO blood groups.
3.   Tissue typing

Cadaveric Donor Kidney
      Donor kidneys are obtained from patients between 10 and 65 years of age who have been admitted to hospital after a sudden catastrophe and in whom recovery is impossible and death is imminent.
      Suitable donors include patients involved in or suffering from:
1.   Major road traffic accidents.
2.   Myocardial infarcts.
3.   Intracranial haemorrhage.
4.   Intracranial tumours.
5.   Pulmonary embolism.
      Permission for removal of the kidneys is obtained from the nearest relative and the coroner before clinical brain death has been verified. The procedure is facilitated in those patients who carry kidney donor cards. The kidneys are removed by an experienced surgeon—usually a member of the renal transplant team.

Survival of Donor Kidney
      Survival of the donor kidney is dependent on the length of ischaemia and is markedly improved by cooling. The removed donor kidney is stored in a plastic container, surrounded by crushed ice at 5 °C. Alternatively, the renal artery may be perfused by a hypothermic albumin solution (*Fig.* 11.3). Total ischaemic time is composed of two factors:
      Warm ischaemia:
          Time between removal of the kidney and cooling to 4 °C. This ischaemic period should not exceed 1 hr.
      Cold ischaemia:
          Time between cooling and implantation of kidney into recipient. This period should not exceed 4 days.
      The donor's blood group and tissue type are ascertained. Incompatibility can be recognized by culturing the donor's and the recipient's lymphocytes. The cooled perfused kidney may be transported to other centres in the UK or Europe if a suitable recipient is available, and provided the transplantation operation can be performed within 4 days of removal of the cadaveric kidney. With this in mind, a computerized kidney bank has been established for the use of European renal transplant centres.

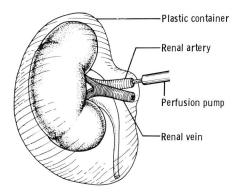

Fig. 11.3 Cooling of a cadaveric kidney by perfusion with an albumin solution at 4 °C.

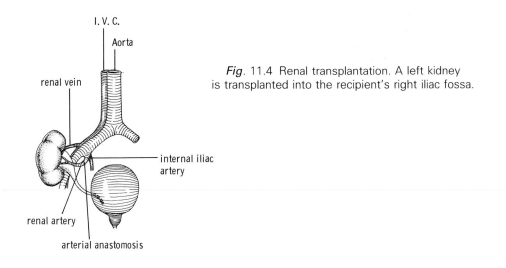

Fig. 11.4 Renal transplantation. A left kidney is transplanted into the recipient's right iliac fossa.

Operation of Renal Transplantation

The donor kidney is transplanted into the iliac fossa of the recipient, the renal artery anastomosed end-to-end with the internal iliac artery, the renal vein anastomosed end-to-side with the external iliac vein and the ureter implanted into the bladder (*Fig*. 11.4).

Postoperative Management of the Transplant

All patients are treated by immunosuppressive therapy in the post-operative period. A combination of azothiaprine (Imuran) and prednisone in large doses is prescribed until the graft is fully functional. Cyclosporin-A is a newer immunosuppressive agent favoured in some centres. The grafted kidney starts to

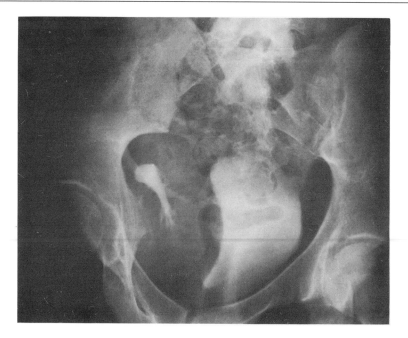

Fig. 11.5 IVU—functional transplanted kidney in right side of pelvis.

function in 3–5 days. When full renal function has been restored, the patient is managed on maintenance immunosuppressive therapy for the life of the grafted kidney. Function of the transplanted kidney is monitored by regular haematological and biochemical estimations and by DMSA scans or an IVU (*Fig.* 11.5) each year.

Complications of Renal Transplantation
1. Infection (bacterial and fungal):
    40 per cent—prompt antibiotic therapy.
2. Cardiovascular and cerebral thrombosis:
    25 per cent—accounts for one-third of deaths after transplantation.
3. Pulmonary embolus:
    Common—anticoagulant therapy.
4. Gastro-intestinal haemorrhage:
    Due to acute peptic ulceration—transfusion.
5. Diabetes:
    Due to steroid therapy.
6. Hypercalcaemia:
    Secondary hyperparathyroidism—subtotal parathyroidectomy.
7. Development of malignancy:
    7 per cent—due to immunosuppression.
8. Mechanical complications:
    Vascular anastomotic leakage—re-operation.
    Leakage from ureteric re-implantation—re-operation.

9.   Rejection crisis:
         Pyrexia, oliguria and occasionally haematuria.
         Immediate treatment by large doses of prednisone.

Results of Renal Transplantation
1.   Mortality rate of operation:
         5–8 per cent.
2.   Mortality rate and later mortality from sepsis or vascular complications:
         25 per cent.
3.   Live donors—recipients of related living allografts:
         60 per cent of kidneys survive 5 years.
4.   Cadaveric grafts:
         40 per cent rejection in first year.
         50 per cent of grafts viable and functioning at 5 years.

Future Trends
         Availability of better quality donor kidneys, improved methods of storage of cadaveric kidneys and development of new immunosuppressive agents are all factors which should contribute to reduction in both morbidity and mortality in the recipient and to prolongation of the functional life of the transplanted kidney.

Index